Keio University International Symposia
for Life Sciences and Medicine 10

Springer

Tokyo
Berlin
Heidelberg
New York
Hong Kong
London
Milan
Paris

J. Kanzaki, M. Tos,
M. Sanna, D.A. Moffat,
T. Kunihiro, Y. Inoue (Eds.)

Acoustic Neuroma

Consensus on Systems for Reporting Results

With 49 Figures

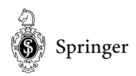 Springer

Jin Kanzaki, M.D.
Professor Emeritus, Department of Otolaryngology, School of Medicine,
Keio University, 35 Shinanomachi, Shinjuku-ku, Tokyo 160-8582, Japan

Mirko Tos, M.D., DMSc dr.h.c.
Professor, Department of Otolaryngology, Gentofte University Hospital,
DK-2900 Hellerup, Denmark

Mario Sanna, M.D.
Professor, Gruppo Otologico Piacenza, Casa di Cura, Via Emmanueli, 42,
29100 Piacenza, Italy

David A. Moffat, M.D.
Professor and Chairman, Department of Otoneurological and Skull Base Surgery,
Addenbrooke's Hospital, Cambridge University Teaching Hospitals Trust, Box 163,
Hills Road, Cambridge, CB2 2QQ, UK

Takanobu Kunihiro, M.D.
Assistant Professor, Department of Otolaryngology, School of Medicine,
Keio University, 35 Shinanomachi, Shinjuku-ku, Tokyo 160-8582, Japan

Yasuhiro Inoue, M.D.
Assistant Professor, Department of Otolaryngology, School of Medicine,
Keio University, 35 Shinanomachi, Shinjuku-ku, Tokyo 160-8582, Japan

ISBN 4-431-70341-1 Springer-Verlag Tokyo Berlin Heidelberg New York
Library of Congress Cataloging-in-Publication Data applied for.
Printed on acid-free paper

Typesetting: SNP Best-set Typesetter Ltd., Hong Kong
Printing and binding: Shinano, Incorporated, Japan
SPIN: 10833023

Foreword

This volume of the Keio University International Symposia for Life Sciences and Medicine contains the proceedings of the eleventh symposium held under the sponsorship of the Keio University Medical Science Fund. As explained in the Opening Remarks by the President of Keio University, the fund was established by the generous donation of Dr. Mitsunada Sakaguchi. The Keio University International Symposia for Life Sciences and Medicine constitute one of the core activities sponsored by the fund, the objective of which is to contribute to the international community by developing human resources, promoting scientific knowledge, and encouraging mutual exchange. Each year, the Committee of the International Symposia for Life Sciences and Medicine selects the most significant symposium topic from applications received from the Keio medical community. The publication of the proceedings is intended to publicize and disseminate the information arising from the lively discussions of the most exciting and current issues presented during the symposium. On behalf of the Committee, I am most grateful to Dr. Mitsunada Sakaguchi, who made the symposia series possible. We are also grateful to the prominent speakers for their contribution to this volume. In addition, we would like to acknowledge the efficient organizational work performed by the members of the program committee and the staff of the fund.

Naoki Aikawa, M.D., D.M.Sc., F.A.C.S.
Chairman
Committee of the International Symposia
for Life Sciences and Medicine

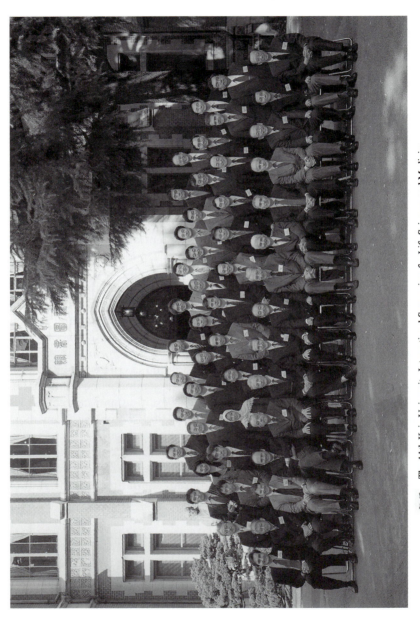

The 11th Keio University International Symposium for Life Sciences and Medicine
Consensus Meeting on Systems for Reporting Results in Acoustic Neuroma   *November 7-9, 2001*

Preface

Dear Colleagues:

We are pleased to convene a meeting of leading world experts to discuss and to reach a consensus on "Systems for Reporting Results in Acoustic Neuroma," the title of the 11th Keio University International Symposium for Life Sciences and Medicine in the very first year of the twenty-first century.

The number of surgical and nonsurgical reports on acoustic neuroma has increased as the existence of this specific tumor has been recognized through the widespread use of magnetic resonance imaging (MRI). It is often difficult, however, to make inter-institutional comparisons of reports because the data are presented in different forms. Results on the treatment or management of acoustic neuroma should be reported through systems that are internationally accepted by standardized evaluation methods. Reporting systems which we hope will be used internationally should provide a standard that will be adopted for inter-institutional comparison of results after surgery or radiosurgery and for clinical purposes. Therefore, the systems should be simple, easy to remember, and easy to use, to facilitate comparison of the results from one institution with those from another. We may be able to use two reporting systems, one an international system for comparing results among researchers, the other a reporting system for academic purposes, to be used mainly within a given country. All of us have already used a reporting system of our own. That may be more convenient to use in some situations, such as domestic congresses. Even in such cases, we have to prepare a method to translate our own reporting system into an international one.

The importance of the standardization of reporting results was stated in an editorial of the *American Journal of Otology* in 1996, and reporting standards for grading of facial nerve function (House-Brackmann's grading system) and hearing preservation after acoustic neuroma surgery were adopted by that journal.

The importance of the standardization of reporting results has been emphasized since the first acoustic neuroma conference in Copenhagen, held in 1991. At the recent conference on acoustic neuroma in Rome, in June 1999, reporting systems were discussed. However, as always, the main problem is that the time allotted to talk about these systems in a conference is too short. Under these circumstances, it seems difficult to propose a standard reporting system, especially as the acoustic neuroma conference is held only once every 4 years. Considering this situation, we planned to hold the consensus meeting with the financial support of the Keio University Medical Science Fund, with the agreement of the past presidents and the president-elect. Fortunately, during the early planning of this meeting, we obtained the agreement of many surgeons involved in acoustic neuroma surgery, because they all recognized the importance of the nature of the meeting. As distinguished members who participated in the past three international acoustic neuroma conferences have kindly accepted our invitation to contribute to internationally accepted reporting systems in acoustic neuroma surgery, I am convinced that this unique meeting will be both exciting and successful.

Jin Kanzaki, M.D.

Chairman, 11th Keio University International Symposium for Life Sciences and Medicine, Consensus Meeting on Systems for Reporting Results in Acoustic Neuroma
Professor and Chairman, Department of Otolaryngology, School of Medicine, Keio University, Tokyo

Contents

Part 6   Summaries of Meeting Sessions

List of Contributors

Opening Remarks

Professor Yuichiro Anzai
President, Keio University
Chairman, Keio University Medical Science Fund

Distinguished guests, ladies and gentlemen; Dr. Tos, President of the first international conference on acoustic neuroma in 1991; Dr. Charachon, President of the second conference in 1995; Dr. Sanna, President of the third conference in 1999; and Dr. Moffat, President of the fourth conference in 2003.

On behalf of Keio University, it is a great pleasure to welcome all of you to the 11th Keio University International Symposium for Life Sciences and Medicine. I am particularly grateful to the distinguished medical scientists who have traveled such long distances to participate in this meeting.

The major subject of this year's symposium is "Systems for Reporting Results in Acoustic Neuroma."

Although remarkable progress and breakthroughs are reported almost every day in the research field of skull base surgery, it is also true that there are still some patients who suffer in spite of surgery and radiotherapy. In this regard, I believe that it is an opportune time to hold a symposium at Keio University related to the subject. All speakers kindly accepted our invitation to contribute to this symposium on systems for reporting results in acoustic neuroma, and I feel certain that this unique meeting will prove both exciting and successful.

Keio was founded in 1858 by Yukichi Fukuzawa and is the oldest university in the country. Fukuzawa was a pioneer in the modernization of Japan. He was a member of the very first mission of the Tokugawa Shogunate government to the United States in 1860 and to European countries in 1862. Before that time, Japan's doors to the outside world had been closed in a period of self-isolationism lasting almost 300 years. Fukuzawa realized during his visits to the United States and Europe that education and learning were crucially important and inevitable in the future of Japan. Keio has its origins in international exchanges; indeed, international exchanges such as this symposium have been one of the most important academic and social missions of Keio University since its foundation.

In the fall of 1994, Dr. Mitsunada Sakaguchi, an alumnus of the class of 1940 of our medical school, donated five billion yen, approximately 40 million dollars, to the university. He expressed the wish that his fund be used to encourage research in life sciences and medicine and to promote worldwide advancements in life sciences. We agreed with his proposal and thus launched the Keio University Medical Science Fund in April 1995. The International Symposia for Life Sciences and Medicine have been organized as one of several projects supported by the fund. In 1999, Dr. Sakaguchi made an additional donation of two billion yen. With these funds, Keio University now plans to start a new laboratory in the field of life sciences and medicine.

It is thus more than a pleasure, indeed it is an honor, for me to be able to meet the distinguished medical researchers and clinicians from world-renowned institutions who kindly gathered here, and to share in frank and valuable exchanges of views. I am also grateful for the efforts made by the organizing committee, chaired by Dr. Jin Kanzaki, who has devoted himself to ensuring that this symposium is an auspicious and enjoyable event. I do hope that the meeting will prove a truly fruitful and productive one for you all.

Let me close by wishing everyone gathered here further success in your research and clinical work. Thank you very much.

Part 1
Tumor Size

Proposal for Reporting Size of Vestibular Schwannoma

MIRKO TOS and JENS THOMSEN

Summary. Analysis of surgical and epidemiological series as well as wait-and-scan series supports the proposal of the following classification of vestibular schwannomas based on the largest extrameatal diameter only: intrameatal tumors, small tumors (1–10 mm extrameatal size), medium tumors (11–20 mm extrameatal size), large tumors (21–40 mm extrameatal size), and giant tumors (41 mm extrameatal size or larger). We do, however, gladly support the proposal of the Kanzaki group to split large tumors into a group of moderately larger tumors of 21–30 mm extrameatal size and a group of large tumors of 31–40 mm extrameatal size, thus resulting in six size groups.

Key words. Vestibular schwannoma size, Vestibular schwannoma classification, Acoustic neuroma size, Acoustic neuroma classification

Introduction

In the synopsis on disagreements on tumor size at the First International Conference on Acoustic Neuroma in Copenhagen in 1991, we summarized various classifications being used at this conference [1] and proposed a classification of tumor size of acoustic neuroma [2], partly based on the original House classification [3] and partly on our epidemiological classification [4], which included a group of small tumors.

ENT Department, Gentofte University Hospital, DK-2900 Hellerup, Denmark

Our Current Tumor Classification

In our previous as well as in our current tumor classification, intrameatal tumors were clearly distinguished from extrameatal tumors and the largest extrameatal diameter in millimeters (mm) was applied.

From 1975 to 1990, we used the House classification [3], dividing the tumors into small (i.e., intrameatal) tumors, medium tumors with the largest extrameatal diameter 1–25 mm, large tumors measuring 26–40 mm, and giant tumors with an extrameatal diameter larger than 40 mm.

It soon became obvious that a separate group of small extrameatal tumors was necessary, and since 1990 we have used the current classification of vestibular schwannoma (Table 1) in all our publications, dividing the extrameatal tumors into small (1–10 mm), medium (11–25 mm), large (26–40 mm), and giant tumors (with a diameter larger than 40 mm).

In our epidemiological studies, we have used this classification since 1984 [4,5]. The need for a classification of small extrameatal tumors is best illustrated in Table 2, showing the increasing number of small tumors diagnosed in Denmark [6], especially during the most recent period (Table 2).

In our translabyrinthine series we have had only 5 intrameatal tumors, but 102 small extrameatal tumors, which is also a strong argument for a separate

TABLE 1. Classification of vestibular schwannoma applied in 1990 and proposed change of this classification

Used since 1990		Proposed	
Intrameatal		Intrameatal	
Small	1–10 mm	Small	1–10 mm
Medium	11–25 mm	Medium	11–20 mm
Large	26–40 mm	Large	21–40 mm
Giant	>40 mm	Giant	>40 mm

TABLE 2. Number of vestibular schwannomas diagnosed in Denmark during the three periods

			Extrameatal size (mm)				
Period	Years	Intrameatal	Small (1–10)	Medium (11–25)	Large (26–40)	Giant (>40)	Total
July 1976–June 1983	7	1	37	71	68	101	278
July 1983–June 1990	7	1	71	97	95	73	337
July 1990–Dec. 1995	5.5	28	103	112	68	44	355
Total	19.5	30	211	280	231	218	970

From [6], with permission

TABLE 3. Distribution of various sizes of vestibular schwannomas in seven consecutive series including all vestibular schwannomas in Denmark operated on by translabyrinthine approach from March 1976 to December 1995

Consecutive series	Intrameatal	Extrameatal size (mm)				x^2-test
		1–10	11–25	26–40	>40	
1–100	1	20	22	25	32	$P < 0.05$
101–200	0	9	26	25	40	$P < 0.05$
201–300	0	6	16	39	39	$P < 0.05$
301–400	0	14	28	29	29	$P > 0.05$
401–500	0	11	38	29	22	$P > 0.05$
501–600	0	19	34	31	16	$P > 0.05$
601–703	4	23	36	21	16	
Total	5	102	200	199	197	

group of small extrameatal tumors (Table 3). The high number of giant tumors supports our classification with separation of these tumors into a discrete group, even though their number has decreased significantly in recent years (Table 3). The reason for the high number of giant tumors in our series is that we have operated on all acoustic neuromas by the translabyrinthine approach, in particular the larger ones, from all of Denmark (with 5.1 million inhabitants) (Tables 2, 3).

The Proposed Classification

During recent years the "wait-and-scan" management of vestibular schwannomas up to an extrameatal size of 20 mm, especially in elderly patients, has been accepted in Denmark. In this period many intrameatal tumors have been diagnosed and most allocated to wait-and-scan (Table 4). Because of wait-and-scan management many patients with medium-sized tumors are waiting for surgery until the tumors reach an extrameatal size of 20 mm. Therefore, we propose changing our classification in a group of medium tumors with 11–20 mm extrameatal diameter (see Table 1).

A detailed classification of tumor sizes in several size groups is also necessary for a better calculation of risk for postoperative facial nerve palsy, which strongly depends on the size of the tumors [7] (Table 5).

TABLE 4. Number of acoustic neuromas diagnosed in the 5½-year period July 1990 to December 1995 allocated to various surgeries or wait-and-scan treatment

Surgery/ wait-and-scan	Intrameatal	Extrameatal extension (mm)				Total
		Small (0–10)	Medium (11–25)	Large (26–40)	Giant (>40)	
Translabyrinthine	—	53	76	64	44	237
Suboccipital	—	9	13	3	—	25
Middle fossa	2	8	3	—	—	13
Wait-and-scan	26	33	20	1	—	80
Total	28	103	112	68	44	355

From [6], with permission

TABLE 5. Facial nerve function 1 year after translabyrinthine removal of 692 vestibular schwannomas [House–Brackmann (HB) classification]

Facial nerve, HB	Intrameatal, n = 05 (%)	Extrameatal (mm)				Total	
		Small (1–10), n = 102 (%)	Medium (11–25), n = 198 (%)	Large (26–40), n = 190 (%)	Giant (>40), n = 190 (%)	n	%
1	100	81	75	53	32	403	58
2	0	11	12	18	9	88	13
3	0	3	7	12	11	61	9
4	0	0	2	4	9	30	4
5	0	4	2	4	9	33	5
6	0	1	2	8	29	77[a]	11
Total	100	100	100	100	100	692	100

[a] Thirty-five patients with disruption of the facial nerve included
Kruskal–Wallis test: $P < 0.00001$
From [7], with permission

A classification of extrameatal size in 10-mm intervals, by splitting the large-tumor classification (21–40 mm, see Table 1) into two groups of 21–30 mm and 31–40 mm, as suggested by the Kanzaki group [8], has our support. Such classification will be: intrameatal tumors, small tumors (1–10 mm), medium tumors (11–20 mm), moderately large tumors (21–30 mm), large tumors (31–40 mm), and giant tumors (more than 40 mm).

References

1. Tos M, Thomsen J (1992) Synopsis on disagreements in measuring tumor size at the Copenhagen Acoustic Neuroma Conference. In: Tos M, Thomsen J (eds) Acoustic neuroma. Kugler, Amsterdam, pp 995–998

2. Tos M, Thomsen J (1992) Proposal of classification of tumor size in acoustic neuroma surgery. In: Tos M, Thomsen J (eds) Acoustic neuroma. Kugler, Amsterdam, pp 133–137
3. House WF, Luetje CM (1979) Acoustic tumors, vol 2. University Park Press, Baltimore, pp 1–50
4. Tos M, Thomsen J (1984) Epidemiology of acoustic neuromas. J Laryngol Otol 98: 685–692
5. Tos M, Thomsen J, Charabi S (1992) Epidemiology of acoustic neuromas: has the incidence increased during the last years. In: Tos M, Thomsen J (eds) Acoustic neuroma. Kugler, Amsterdam, pp 3–6
6. Tos M, Charabi S, Thomsen J (1999) Incidence of vestibular schwannoma. Laryngoscope 109:736–740
7. Tos M, Charabi S, Thomsen J (1998) Clinical experience with vestibular schwannomas: epidemiology, symptomatology, diagnosis and surgical results. Eur Arch Otolaryngol 255:1–6
8. Kanzaki J, Inoue Y, Kunihiro T (2001) Measurement of tumor size. Keio J Med 50(suppl 4):19

Proposal for Reporting on Size and Site of Residual Vestibular Schwannoma

Mirko Tos and Jens Thomsen

Summary. There is a great need for classification of the size and site of residual tumors deliberately left at the time of surgery for vestibular schwannoma and at regular follow-up by CT or MRI scan. We propose describing the size as the longest and perpendicular diameters of the residuum, e.g., 2×1 mm, 3×2 mm, 4×3 mm, or 10×5 mm. To describe the site of the residuum, we propose to distinguish between (a) in the fundus, (b) in the meatus, (c) around the porus, (d) along the extrameatal nerves, or (e) at the brainstem or the cerebellum. The measurement should also be performed during the first postoperative days by CT or MRI scan and should be repeated at regular intervals.

Key words. Residual vestibular schwannomas, Classification of size of vestibular schwannomas, Classification of site of residual vestibular schwannomas, Residual acoustic neuroma classification

"Wait-and scan" management of vestibular schwannomas (VS) has become an accepted treatment, and today most patients with diagnosed intrameatal, small, or even medium-sized tumors with an extrameatal diameter less than 20 mm require proof that their tumors will grow. Wait-and-scan treatment has resulted in an increasing number of patients with diagnosed VS having repeated magnetic resonance imaging (MRI) scans until it is agreed with the patient that an operation is necessary, usually if the tumor grows toward the 20-mm extrameatal size.

Accepting the wait-and-scan management of VS up to 20 mm extrameatal size, and an even larger size in elderly patients, we should also accept the concept of deliberately leaving a residual piece of tumor at surgery to dimin-

ENT Department, Gentofte University Hospital, DK-2900 Hellerup, Denmark

ish the risk of postoperative sequelae, especially facial nerve palsy. Such treatment for elderly patients was proposed by Silverstein et al. in 1985 [1]. The size and location of residual tumors should be accurately described at surgery, verified with MRI scan postoperatively, and the eventual growth followed by MRI scans at regular intervals.

The following sizes and locations to be registered are proposed:

1. Description of the size of the residuum at surgery; the longest and the perpendicular diameters of the residual tumors are used, e.g., 2×1 mm, 3×2 mm, 4×3 mm, 10×5 mm.
   Description of location of the residual tumor:
   a. In the fundus
   b. In the meatus
   c. Around the porus
   d. Along the extrameatal part of the facial nerve
   e. At the brainstem or the cerebellum, including attachment to the AICA or the trigeminal nerve, the jugular nerve, or the facial nerve
2. Computed tomography (CT) or MRI scans during the first postoperative days, applying the described classification on size and site
3. CT or MRI scans at various intervals, applying the same classification of size as for nonoperated tumors, such as:
   Intrameatal tumors, exclusively intrameatal
   Small tumors, 1–10 mm extrameatal in largest diameter
   Medium tumors, 11–20 mm extrameatal size
   Moderately large tumors, 21–30 mm extrameatal size
   Large tumors, 31–40 mm extrameatal size

The length of the intervals between scans depends on the initial size and location of the residual tumor, age of the patient, and the growth rate of the tumor. In an elderly patient with a small intrameatal residual tumor and slow growth, the intervals could be more than 1 year, whereas in younger patients with growth of the residuum at the brainstem the intervals should be shorter.

Such classification will be useful in multicentric studies. In fact, very little is known about residual tumor after surgery. There appear to be no systematic studies on the features of the residuum. At the First Acoustic Neuroma Conference in Copenhagen in 1991, several reports on near-total, subtotal, or partial removal of acoustic neuromas were discussed and presented, showing that some residual tumors do not grow [2–5].

In our series of 703 patients operated on for VS using the translabyrinthine approach, we have left small remnants in 1.9% of moderately large tumors with a preoperative extrameatal diameter of 21–30 mm. Among large tumors with a preoperative extrameatal diameter of 31–40 mm, the percentage of residual tumors was 6.5%, and in giant tumors it was 16.3%. We have

TABLE 1. Partial tumor removal and leaving small remnants of tumors in 703 patients with vestibular schwannoma by translabyrinthine surgery from July 1976 to December 1994

Extrameatal size (mm)	Total tumors	Partial removal	Small remnants	Total No.	Total %
Intrameatal (0 mm)	5			0	
1–10	105			0	
11–20	153			0	
21–30	157		3	3	1.9
31–40	77		5	5	6.5
>40	9	9[a]			
>40	185	5[b]	18	32	16.3
Total	703	14	26	40	6.3

[a] Planned two-stage operation (translabyrinthine, suboccipital) in 1976–1978 (9 cases)
[b] Reoperated by translabyrinthine approach after 1978 (4 cases)

reoperated by translabyrinthine approach in some cases but have not yet completed our follow-up studies on growth of the residual tumors. We are, however, not aware of any deaths caused by the residual tumors. It is our intention to publish the results of a systematic follow-up of all patients with residual tumors (Table 1).

References

1. Silverstein H, McDaniels A, Norrell H, et al (1985) Conservative management of acoustic neuroma in the elderly patient. Laryngoscope 95:766–770
2. Moffat DA, Hardy DG (1992) Near-total, subtotal or partial removal of acoustic neuromas. In: Tos M, Thomsen J (eds) Acoustic neuroma. Kugler, Amsterdam, pp 691–696
3. Kemink JL, Tucci DL, Telian SA, et al (1992) Near-total and subtotal resection of acoustic neuroma. In: Tos M, Thomsen J (eds) Acoustic neuroma. Kugler, Amsterdam, pp 697–700
4. Gamache FW Jr, Patterson RH Jr (1992) Growth rates for residual and recurrent acoustic neuroma. In: Tos M, Thomsen J (eds) Acoustic neuroma. Kugler, Amsterdam, pp 705–707
5. Moffat DA (1992) Synopsis on near-total, subtotal or partial removal. In: Tos M, Thomsen J (eds) Acoustic neuroma. Kugler, Amsterdam, pp 983–984

Classification of Vestibular Schwannoma (Acoustic Neuroma)

SHO HASHIMOTO

Summary. To improve the understanding of acoustic neuromas and to compare the results of their management, the same reporting system must be used in each subject. Tumor size and location are very important for preoperative assessment of tumor characteristics. Tumors should be classified into four categories: intrameatal (IM), small (S), medium (M), and large (L). The IM tumor is limited to the internal auditory meatus. The S tumor is up to 15mm in extrameatal size, the M tumor is more than 15mm and no more than 30mm, and the L tumor is more than 30mm. The actual tumor size should be noted as [maximum diameter] × [minimum diameter]. When hearing preservation is attempted, the status of the fundus may be critical. If the fundus is occupied by the tumor, the tumor must be removed by blind dissection, and the cochlear nerve at its most vulnerable part as well as the vessels will be damaged, which results in the failure of hearing preservation. Therefore the status of the fundus should be stated together with the tumor size: e.g., IM, fundus occupied, or M 28 × 24, fundus empty.

Key words. Fundus, Hearing preservation, MRI

Introduction

To improve the understanding of acoustic neuromas and to compare the results of their management, the same reporting system must be used in each subject. Tumor size and location are very important for preoperative assessment of tumor characteristics. Each category of classification should reflect the tumor characteristics, such as compression of the nerves, brainstem, or

Department of Otolaryngology, National Sendai Hospital, 2-8-8 Miyagino, Miyagino-ku, Sendai 983-8520, Japan cerebellum. The classification should also be easy to understand and to remember so that many doctors will use it. In this chapter, concepts of a classification based on surgical anatomy are proposed and discussed.

Classification of Size

The author has classified tumors into four categories[1]; intra-meatal(IM), small(S), medium(M), and large(L). The IM tumor is limited to the internal auditory meatus. The S tumor is up to 15mm in extrameatal size, the M tumor is more than 15mm and no more than 30mm, and the L tumor is more than 30mm. The size of the intrameatal portion of S, M, and L tumors should not be included in the measurement, because it has no meaning in the management of the disease. No matter how large the intrameatal portion is, the operation is not affected and the possibility of functional preservation is not different. The only issue in the internal auditory meatus that will influence the results of management is whether the fundus is invaded by the tumor; this question will be discussed later.

In the IM tumor (Fig. 1), the nerves are compressed between the meatal wall and the tumor but are never bent at the porus acousticus internus. With few exceptions, adhesion between the tumor and the nerves is not severe, and the tumor is easily dissected from the nerves without damaging them.

The S tumor often touches the brainstem but is not adherent to it, because the length of the 8th nerve between the brainstem and the porus is around

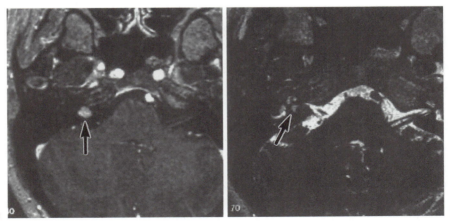

FIG. 1. Vestibular schwannoma, intrameatal (IM), fundus empty. **a** MRI, T1-weighted image with gadolinium. Tumor (*arrow*) is limited to the internal auditory meatus. **b** Constructive interference in steady state (CISS) image. Fluid space (*arrow*) is seen at the fundus. Nerves are recognized in the meatus of the opposite side. The tumor was removed by the retrosigmoid approach and hearing was well preserved with 5 dB gain

15 mm[2] . It compresses the nerves in the meatus and at the porus, but the nerve root at the brainstem is not compressed by the S tumor. Adhesion to the nerves is most severe at the porus, where the nerves are bent and funning of them is usually seen. This is the most dangerous part of nerve damage, and the procedure must be undertaken most carefully at this point in the removal of the tumor of this category.

The M tumor compresses the nerve root but does not cause cerebellar signs in many cases. However, because there may be adhesion to the nerve root and brainstem with stretching of the nerves, hearing preservation is usually difficult in this category.

The L tumor, which measures more than 30 mm, often causes brainstem and cerebellum compression that results in cerebellar signs such as unsteadiness and ataxia. Hearing preservation is impossible in the vast majority of cases in this category, and most attention should be paid to preservation of facial function.

Direction of Measurement

The author used to measure the tumor along the axis of the internal auditory meatus as described above, but later the method was changed to measurement of the maximum diameter at the same time, because it has become clear that the tumors tend to grow more in the direction parallel to the petrous ridge. Thus, the actual tumor size should be noted as [maximum diameter] × [minimum diameter]. The classification may be based on the maximum diameter, because the difficulty of management is predicted by the maximum diameter.

Fundus

When hearing preservation is attempted, the status of the fundus of the internal auditory meatus may be critical. The fundus is divided into upper and lower parts by the transverse crest. The lower part is further divided into the pars vestibularis and the pars cochlearis. The latter usually forms cupping where many small holes form the spiral shape, through which the nerve fibers enter the modiolus of the cochlea. The author calls this part the "cochlear fundus." The fluid space and the nerves at the fundus are well visualized by heavily T2-weighted MRI images, especially by constructive interference in steady state (CISS) MRI [3] (Fig. 2).

The cochlear nerve consists of thousands of nerve fibers that are divided into nerve fascicles at the cochlear fundus and enter the modiolus of the cochlea. This is the most vulnerable part of the cochlear nerve and should not be disturbed during surgery. However, the cochlear fundus can never be

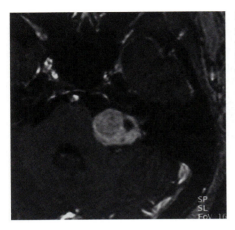

FIG. 2. Vestibular schwannoma, M 28 × 24 mm, fundus empty. MRI, T1-weighted image with gadolinium. The tumor was removed by the retrosigmoid approach and hearing was preserved

observed through the middle fossa approach because of the overhanging transverse crest. It also cannot be observed through the retrosigmoid approach because of the vestibule and the posterior semicircular canal. If the fundus is occupied by the tumor, the tumor must be removed by blind dissection and the cochlear nerve as well as the vessels will be damaged, which results in the failure of hearing preservation. Therefore, the status of the fundus should be stated together with the tumor size: IM, fundus occupied, or S13 × 11, fundus empty, etc.

Conclusion

The classification of vestibular schwannoma must be simple and easy to understand so that it will be used worldwide. Each category should describe the characteristics of the included tumor. The state of the cochlear fundus must be noted so that the possibility of hearing preservation can be predicted.

References

1. Hashimoto S (1991) MR imaging in the diagnosis and treatment of acoustic neuromas. In: Tos M, Thomsen J (eds) Acoustic neuroma. Kugler Publications, Amsterdam, pp 141–144
2. Lang J (1991) Clinical anatomy of the posterior cranial fossa and its foramina. Georg Thieme, New York, pp 83–91
3. Casselman JW, et al (1996) Constructive interference in steady state-3DFT MR imaging of the inner ear and cerebellopontine angle. AJNR 17:1099–1105

The Size of the Tumor in Acoustic Neuroma: Proposal for a Reporting System

Miguel Arístegui

Summary. Determining the size of the tumor in acoustic neuroma is essential because the size influences preoperative assessment, patient outcome, amount of tumor removal, and follow-up of residual tumor, after radiotherapy, and scan-and-see policy. Until a reliable method to determine the volume of the tumor is established and widely used, we should adopt a simple one that allows comparison of different series. A proposal of such a method is described. The intracanalicular (IC) and extracanalicular (EC) parts of the tumor should be measured separately and the largest dimension of each reported. A parallel classification is added that includes several characteristics of the tumor that are not defined by a number. The suggested method is a simple one that could be applied to previous series, and easily adopted for future ones, until an accurate volume tracing method exists and is widely used.

Key words. Acoustic neuroma, Size, Measurements, Reporting system, Follow-up

Introduction

Great discrepancy exists between different authors in the assessment of tumor size. We are all speaking about small, medium, large, or giant tumors, and there is no agreement about the size of the tumor for each group. Linear measurements are the most widely used, with area tracing methods and volume tracing methods being proposed as more accurate. Unfortunately, we are still not close to 100% accuracy, and no new method has gained advocates. Until

Servicio ORL, Hospital Central Cruz Roja, Avda. Reina Victoria, 26, 28003 Madrid, Spain

a reliable and accurate method based on computer technology exists, we should keep a more easily adopted linear method that allows comparison between different series. A method easily adapted for other linear methods, in which quantitative and qualitative aspects of intracanicular (IC) and extra-canalicular (EC) tumors are reported separately, is proposed.

Materials

Proceedings of the three International Meetings on Acoustic Neuromas held in Copenhagen in 1991, Paris in 1995, and Rome in 1999 have been reviewed to observe the discrepancy between different groups of surgeons in assessing the size of the tumor and the subdivision in subgroups of different sizes.

Results

In all three publications of the international meetings on acoustic neuromas, we see many different ways of reporting the size of the tumor. No agreement is yet present, and it is difficult to find two groups reporting in the same way.

Tos and Thomsen [1] made an excellent synopsis on disagreements in measuring tumor size at the Copenhagen Acoustic Neuroma Conference. The reader is referred to this paper to see the wide range of different classifications. In the same volume, Tos and Thomsen [2] reported their own discrepancy, and showed their previous classification, their current one, and new proposals for discussion.

Discrepancy starts in the way different authors measure the tumor. Alternative descriptors of tumor size include: the whole length of the IC and EC portions of the tumor, the largest EC dimension, the largest EC dimension parallel to the petrous pyramid, the largest EC dimension perpendicular to the pyramid, and the largest dimension in the axis of the internal auditory canal (IAC). Many authors do not describe their method of measurment. Even though area tracing methods or volume-tracing methods are being suggested, nearly all are still using linear methods to measure tumor size. The division between small and medium tumors varies from 1.0 to 2.5 cm, while the division between medium and large tumors varies from 2.0 to 4.0 cm. Most authors use purely numeric values to subdivide groups [2–17], some use anatomic references [IC, no contact with brainstem (BS), contact with BS, displacement of ventricles] [18], and some use a combination [19,20]. Some authors have even changed their method after a time.

Surprisingly, there have been few proposals since the Copenhagen meeting, with few papers including this topic [19,20]. However, the need to reach a consensus still exists.

Discussion

Accurate assessment of the size of acoustic tumors is essential for preoperative evaluation, for reporting results (hearing preservation, facial nerve outcome, complication rate, etc.), for follow-up after radiotherapy, to assess residual tumor, and in the scan-and-see policy to evaluate tumor progression rate. Little agreement exists in however, assessing tumor size and as to what should be considered a small, medium, or large tumor, in spite of its relevance for comparing series from different authors.

Future technology is likely to lead to an accurate volume-tracing method that will give an exact cubic millimeter (mm^3) number that will allow proper comparison among groups of patients. Until that technology is available and universally applied, a linear tracing method, although less accurate, seems to be preferred by almost all authors. Unfortunately, again, disagreement exists in the way such measurement should be obtained. Some include the IC and EC portions in the value and some exclude the IC part. When measuring the EC part of the tumor, some use the largest dimension, some the largest dimension in the axis of the IAC, some the largest dimension parallel to the petrous pyramid, and some the largest perpendicular to it. Figure 1 shows the inadequacy of using the IC portion for measurment; Fig. 2 shows the inadequacy of excluding the IC portion; and Fig. 3 shows how it could also be inadequate to measure parallel or perpendicular to the pyramid, or parallel to the axis of

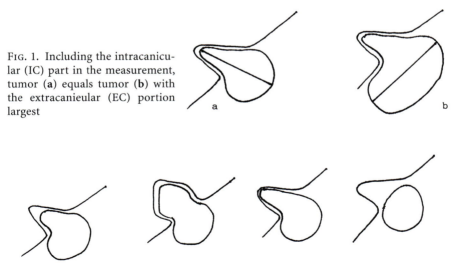

FIG. 1. Including the intracanicular (IC) part in the measurement, tumor (a) equals tumor (b) with the extracanieular (EC) portion largest

FIG. 2. These four tumors were designated as the same by authors who excluded the IC portion from their measurements

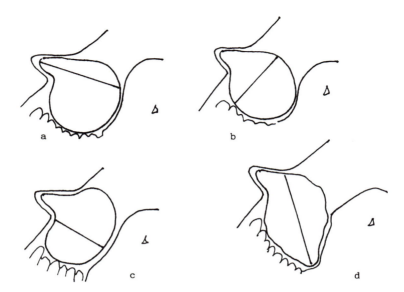

FIG. 3. Measuring the largest dimension in the axis of the internal auditory canal (IAC)
(**a**), parallel (**b**), or perpendicular (**c**) to the petrous pyramid could be inadequate depending on the shape of the tumor. **d** None of the previous measurements are adequate; the
largest EC dimension is more suitable

the IAC. In my experience, the most adequate measurement is the largest EC
dimension. The IC part should be addressed also, but separately, with the
largest IC dimension the most appropriate. Each tumor can be assessed by an
IC number (which could be 0 for medial-type tumors) and an EC number
(which could be 0 for purely IC tumors).

Subdividing different tumor sizes as small, medium, large, and giant could
be awkward in terminology and provide some difficulty in reaching a consensus. Thus, it seems more appropriate to grade tumors into different size
categories where each category spans a range of 10 mm. Table 1 shows such a
proposal; authors could easily find significant differences in results between
different groups without mentioning small, medium, or large, with Grade 1
up to 1 cm, Grade 2 up to 2 cm, etc.

Tumors have characteristics that are difficult to address, such as the shape,
the adherence to neurovascular structures, and the cystic or solid appearance
of the tumor; certainly, these should be descriptive, if necessary. However, the
size of the cerebelo-pontine angle (CPA) is not the same for each patient, and
the relative size of the tumor to the CPA could vary depending not exclusively
on the size of the tumor. Certainly, a 1.0-cm tumor will not touch the BS, but
a 1.5-cm tumor may or may not touch. A 2-cm tumor will touch the BS but
may or may not compress it. A 3-cm tumor will compress the BS but could

TABLE 1. Tumor size grading system

Grade 0:	intracanalicular (0 cm EC)
Grade 1:	0–10 mm EC
Grade 2:	11–20 mm EC
Grade 3:	21–30 mm EC
Grade 4:	31–40 mm EC
Grade 5:	41–50 mm EC
Grade 6:	51–60 mm EC
Grade 7:	61–70 mm EC (etc., if necessary)

EC, extracanicular

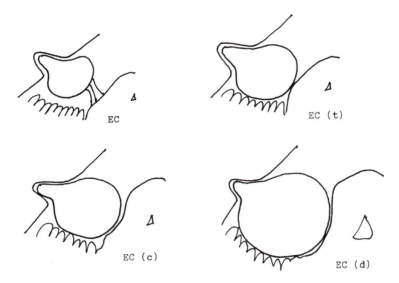

FIG. 4. EC assessment of the tumor: *t*, touching the brainstem (BS); *c*, compressing the BS; *d*, displacing or dilating the ventricular system

dilate the IVth ventricle and may or may not displace it. Thus, it is reasonable to suggest that a letter should be added to the size of the tumor that expresses if the tumor touches the BS (t), compresses the BS (c), or displaces or dilates the ventricular system (d); this letter could thereby subdivide each group of different sizes. Figure 4 shows each EC case. In a similar fashion the IC portion of the tumor should also be given further assessment. A letter should be added to the IC number (in mm), indicating how far there is dilation of the IAC (d), how far the tumor reaches the fundus (f, followed by the number of millimeters of free fundus), or both (d,f) (Fig. 5).

Figure 6 illustrates three examples of the proposed reporting system. A purely IC tumor of 8 mm that dilates the IAC and apparently leaves 2 mm of

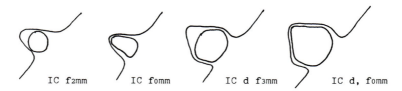

FIG. 5. IC assessment of the tumor: *f*, reaching the fundus (millimeters free); *d*, dilating the IAC. 0 mm for tumors reaching completely the fundus

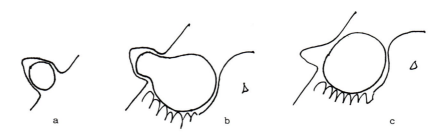

FIG. 6a–c. Three examples of the suggested reporting system. **a** Grade 0: EC 0 mm, IC 8 mm (d,f 2 mm) (intracanalicular type). **b** Grade 2: EC 20 mm, IC 8 mm (d,f 2 mm). **c** Grade 2: EC 20 mm, IC 0 mm (medial-type tumor)

TABLE 2. Tumor removal categories

Total tumor removal:	100%
Near-total removal:	small pieces left
Partial removal:	>50% <100%
Biopsy:	<50%

free fundus, will be grade 0: EC 0 mm, IC 8 mm (d,f 2 mm). A tumor with the same IC portion and an EC portion of 20 mm and compressing the BS will be grade 2: EC 20 mm (c), IC 8 mm (d,f 2 mm). A so-called medial-type tumor without an IC component, and with 2 cm in its EC portion compressing the BS, will be grade 2: EC 20 mm (c), IC 0 mm.

Finally, the degree of tumor resection, should also be addressed, and a proposed system is described as follows: total removal for 100% removal, near-total removal for small pieces of tumor left over the facial, the cochlear, or the BS, partial removal for more than 50% and less than 100% (in cases other than that mentioned in near-total removal), and biopsy for less than 50% removal (Table 2).

Conclusion

A proposal is made for the assessment of tumor size. An IC mm (d,f mm)—EC mm (t,c,d) method, and a grading system for tumor size classification are proposed, which provide a method that is easy to remember for addressing the size of the tumor.

References

1. Tos M, Thomsen J (1992) Synopsis on disagreements in measuring tumor size at the Copenhagen Acoustic Neuroma Conference. In: Acoustic neuroma. Kugler, Amsterdam, pp 975–978
2. Tos M, Thomsen J (1992) Proposals of classification of tumor size in acoustic neuroma surgery. Acoustic neuroma. Kugler, Amsterdam, pp 133–137
3. House WF, Luetje CM (1979) Acoustic tumors, vol 2. University Park Press, Baltimore
4. Glasscock ME III, Levine SC, McKennan KX (1987) The changing characteristics of acoustic neuroma patients over the last ten years. Laryngoscope 97:1164–1167
5. Sterkers O, Badr El Dine M, Martin N, et al (1992) Slow versus rapid growing acoustic neuromas. In: Acoustic neuroma. Kugler, Amsterdam, pp 145–147
6. Pasquier B, Wozniak ZM, Mouret P, et al (1992) Evaluation of the acoustic neuroma growth rate by immunohistological techniques. In: Acoustic neuroma. Kugler, Amsterdam, pp 173–176
7. Noren G, Greitz D, Hirsch A, et al (1992) Gamma knife radiosurgery in acoustic neuromas. In: Acoustic neuroma. Kugler, Amsterdam, pp 289–292
8. Chen JM, Fisch U (1992) The transotic approach in acoustic neuroma surgery. In: Acoustic neuroma. Kugler, Amsterdam, pp 317–323
9. Ekvall L, Kinnefors A, Bynke O, et al (1992) Experience and results in 261 consecutive patients with acoustic tumors operated on with the translabyrinthine technique. In: Acoustic neuroma. Kugler, Amsterdam, pp 347–352
10. Brawanski A, Ullrich OW, Butterhof I, et al (1992) Management of acoustic neuromas in a combined interdisciplinary approach. In: Acoustic neuroma. Kugler, Amsterdam, pp 451–453
11. Kanzaki J, Ogawa K, Shiobara R, et al (1992) Hearing preservation by the extended middle cranial fossa approach for acoustic neuroma. In: Acoustic neuroma. Kugler, Amsterdam, pp 473–477
12. Haid CT, Wigand ME (1992) Surgery of acoustic neuromas via the enlarged middle cranial fossa approach. In: Acoustic neuroma. Kugler, Amsterdam, pp 483–488
13. Dutton JEM, Ramsden R, Lye RH, et al (1992) The neuro-otological team approach to the surgical management of acoustic neuroma: the Manchester experience. In: Acoustic neuroma. Kugler, Amsterdam, pp 503–507
14. Moffat DA, Hardy DG (1992) Near-total, subtotal or partial removal of acoustic neuromas. In: Acoustic neuroma. Kugler, Amsterdam, pp 691–696
15. Walsh RM, Pracy JP, Gleeson MJ, et al (1996) The value of facial nerve monitoring in acoustic tumor surgery. In: Acoustic neuroma and skull base surgery. Kugler, Amsterdam, pp 127–130
16. Mancini F, Falcioni M, Landolfi M, et al (1996) Management of acoustic neuroma through the enlarged translabyrinthine approach. How can we improve the results? In: Acoustic neuroma and skull base surgery. Kugler, Amsterdam, pp 185–193

17. Tanaka Y, Kobayashi S, Hongo K, et al (1999) Radiological analysis of intratumoral cysts in acoustic neuromas. In: Acoustic neuromas and other CPA tumors. Monduzzi, Rome, pp 143–146
18. Bebear JP, Darrouzet V, Guerin J (1992) Acoustic nerve neurinomas: 20 years experience in Bordeaux: 600 cases. In: Acoustic neuroma. Kugler, Amsterdam, pp 517–519
19. Zini C, Magnan J, Piazza F, et al (1999) New anatomo-radio-surgical classification of acoustic neuromas. In: Acoustic neuromas and other CPA tumors. Monduzzi, Rome, pp 117–120
20. Arístegui M (1999) The size of the tumor. Acoustic neuromas and other CPA tumors. Monduzzi, Rome, pp 121–127

Proposal for Definition of Tumor Size

Akira Hara and Jun Kusakari

Summary. The clinical records of 91 cases of acoustic neuroma, operated on at the University Hospital of Tsukuba, were reviewed. In 10 cases with intracanalicular tumor, and 7 cases with a tumor upto 10 mm in diameter, no tumors were found to touch the brainstem in intraoperative findings. Furthermore, in 24 cases with tumor diameter ranging from 11 to 14 mm, no tumors were found touching the brainstem. In 8 cases with a tumor 15–19 mm in diameter, all tumors were touching the brainstem, and symptoms caused by compression of the brainstem were recognized in 6 cases. In 17 cases with a tumor 20–29 mm in diameter, every tumor was found to be adhesive to the brainstem. Every case of 25 acoustic neuroma of 30 mm or more in the largest diameter had symptoms caused by compression of the brainstem, and the tumors were strongly adhesive to the brainstem with no exception. Therefore, we propose this definition of tumor size based on relation to the brainstem: small, from 0 to 14 mm; medium, from 15 to 29 mm; and large, 30 mm or more in the largest diameter of the tumor in the extracanalicular portion.

Key words. Acoustic neuroma, Tumor size, Brainstem, Operation, Medium size

Introduction

The definition of tumor size is very important in acoustic neuroma (AN) preoperative assessment, assessment of tumor growth, post-operative and postirradiation follow-up, and reporting results.Unfortunately, great confusion has existed in reporting methods to assess the tumor size of AN.

Department of Otolaryngology, Institute of Clinical Medicine, University of Tsukuba, 1-1-1 Tennodai, Tsukuba 305-8575, Japan

The Japanese Society of Acoustic Neuroma is now proposing the definition of tumor size as follows: small, from 0 to 10 mm; medium, from 11 to 30 mm; and large, 31 mm or more in the largest diameter of the tumor at the extracanalicular portion. The definition of tumor size should allow that the size diagnostically reported be related to, and reflect, the therapeutic modality and the prognosis. Therefore, to clarify the relation of tumor size and clinical, especially intraoperative, findings, the clinical records of AN cases operated on at our hospital were reviewed.

Materials and Methods

The clinical records of 91 AN cases, operated on at the University Hospital of Tsukuba from June 1988 to May 2001, were reviewed. The operations were performed by the authors (A.H. and/or J.K.) and neurosurgeons using suboccipital, translabyrinthine, or middle cranial fossa approaches. Definitions as to whether the tumor was touching the brainstem and whether the adhesion of the tumor to the brainstem was strong were based on the surgery records.

Results

A summary of the results concerning tumor size and its relation to the brainstem is shown in Table 1. In 10 cases with intracanalicular tumor, and 7 cases with a tumor up to 10 mm in diameter, no tumors were found to touch the brainstem in intraoperative findings. Furthermore, in 24 cases with tumor diameter ranging from 11 to 14 mm, no tumors were touching the brainstem. In contrast, in 8 cases with tumor diameter ranging from 15 to 19 mm, symptoms caused by compression of the brainstem were recognized in 6 cases, and

TABLE 1. Tumor size and its relation to the brainstem

Tumor size[a]	Touching the brainstem	Adhesion to the brainstem	Brainstem symptom[b]	Total
Intracanalicular	0	0	0	10
0–10 mm	0	0	0	7
11–14 mm	0	0	0	24
15–19 mm	8	7	6	8
20–29 mm	17	17	7	17
30 mm or more	25	25	25	25

Numbers represent the number of cases
[a] Tumor size represents the largest diameter of the tumor in millimeters
[b] Acoustic neuroma cases with any symptom caused by compression of the brainstem

every tumor was touching the brainstem. In 17 cases with tumor diameter ranging from 20 to 29 mm, 7 cases had symptoms caused by compression of the brainstem, and every tumor was found to be touching and adhesive to the brainstem. Every case of 25 acoustic neuromas 30 mm or more in the largest diameter had symptoms caused by compression of the brainstem, and the tumors were strongly adhesive to the brainstem with no exception.

Discussion and Conclusion

There are many reporting methods to assess the tumor size of AN [1–3]. In the proposal now made by the Japanese Society of Acoustic Neuroma, the definitions are as follows: small, from 0 to 10 mm; medium, from 11 to 30 mm; and large, 31 mm or more in the largest diameter of the tumor in the extra-canalicular portion. Based on the results of the present study, the definition of a medium-size tumor is controversial. A retrospective study of our AN patients revealed that tumors upto 14 mm in the largest diameter never touched the brainstem in intraoperative findings. When the tumor touches the brainstem or adheres to it, the surgery is difficult and, moreover, surgical outcome is poorer, such as the degree of postoperative facial palsy or preservation of useful hearing. Every tumor of 30 mm or more in the largest diameter was touching and adhesive to the brainstem with no exception, and every AN patient with this size tumor had symptoms caused by compression of the brainstem. Therefore, we would like to propose a definition of tumor size based on its relation to the brainstem: ear tumor; intracanalicular tumor; small, from 0 to 14 mm; medium, from 15 to 29 mm; large, 30 mm or more in the largest diameter of the tumor in the extracanalicular portion [4].

References

1. Pfleiderer AG, Evans KL, Grace ARH, et al (1988) A screening protocol used for the detection of acoustic neuromas: a clinical evaluation. Clin Otolaryngol 13:145–151
2. Clifton AG, Phelps PD, Lloyd GAS (1991) The investigation of acoustic neuroma. Clin Radiol 44:232–235
3. Kusakari J, Kobayashi T, Rokugo M, et al (1984) Diagnosis of acoustic neuroma. J Otorhinolaryngol Jpn 87:923–935
4. Hara A, Ito Z, Wada T, et al (1998) Diagnosis and cost analysis in acoustic neuromas. Otolaryngology (Tokyo) 8:1–5

Classification of Tumor Size from the Point of View of Functional Preservation, Based Upon Our 53 Surgical Cases with Acoustic Neuroma

Kazuo Ishikawa[1], Zhiwei Cao[1], Yan Wang[1], Katsumi Monoo[1], and Nobuyuki Yasui[2]

Summary. The possibility of developing an appropriate classification of tumor size from the point of view of functional preservation was examined from our experience with 53 surgical cases. It was found that almost all the cases considered to be candidates for hearing preservation (and which in fact demonstrated successful postoperative serviceable hearing) were of a tumor size of up to 15 mm from the porus. In addition, it is generally considered that the upper limit of tumor size treatable with radiation is 25 mm, and that hearing preservation can be expected in cases with tumor size up to 25 mm from the porus. In intracanalicular tumor cases, hearing preservation is difficult if the tumor occupies the whole meatus. Thus, the following classification was suggested: intracanalicular tumor (type a, sparing the fundus; type b, occupying the whole meatus), small (0.1–15 mm), medium (15.1–25 mm), large (25.1–35 mm), and giant (35.1 mm or more).

Key words. Acoustic neuroma, Tumor size, Classification, Functional preservation

Introduction

Traditionally, the size of acoustic neuromas and other cerebellopontinoe angle tumors has been measured as the largest diameter from the porus acousticus. However, there is significant confusion in reported size of acoustic neuroma, and no standardized method for measurement has yet been agreed upon. In addition, several nomenclatures are used to categorize the size of the

[1] Department of Otorhinolaryngology, Akita University, School of Medicine, 1-1-1 Hondo, Akita 010-8543, Japan
[2] Department of Neurosurgery, Research Institute of Brain and Vessels of Akita, Akita 010-0874, Japan

tumor, such as grade, stage, and type. This diversity may have been brought about by the recent development of radiological imaging techniques, new treatment options such as the γ knife, new surgical approaches, and the feasibility of the functional preservation of the facial and cochlear nerve. To improve treatment results, it is expected that we can obtain appropriate information and compare the data; therefore, a standard method for measurement should be adopted.

If we consider the treatment of acoustic neuroma from a historical perspective, the goal of the treatment has progressed from saving the patient to determining the size of the tumor, to preserving the facial nerve, and finally to preserving hearing [1]. Thus, entering the 21st century, the goal of the treatment of acoustic neuroma has been raised to the level of functional preservation of not only the facial nerve but also of cochlear function. With this in mind, we have tried to classify the size of the tumor from the aspect of functional preservation, using data from our surgical cases so far.

Materials and Methods

Fifty-three cases of acoustic neuroma operated on during the past 13 years were considered for the present study. Fifty-one cases were unilateral acoustic neuroma and 2 were bilateral cases. Twenty-eight patients were female and 25 were male, with an age distribution of 13–69 years; their average age was 50.2 years.

The tumor sizes ranged from intracanalicular to 45 mm from the porus acousticus (Table 1). Preoperative facial nerve function was normal in all cases. Regarding preoperative hearing acuity, 13 cases were categorized in class A (less than 30 dB of pure tone threshold and more than 70% of speech discrimination), 8 cases in class B (less than 50 dB of pure tone threshold and more than 50% of speech discrimination), 10 cases in class C, and 21 cases in class D according to the AAO-HNS criteria. One case was not fully examined. Regarding postoperative facial nerve function, the House–Brackmann (HB) grading system was used.

As for the surgical approach, 47 cases were via the middle cranial fossa, and in 6 cases with a large tumor we used a combined approach of suboccipital and middle cranial fossa approach.

Results

Anatomic preservation of the facial nerve was obtained in 49 of the 53 cases (92.5%). In 4 cases, the nerve was severed; the tumor sizes were 8, 13, 15, and 31 mm from the porus. In 2 cases, sural nerve grafting was performed, and in the others end-to-end anastomosis. When the final result of facial nerve func-

TABLE 1. Summary of our results of 53 cases

Tumor size		Hearing acuity		Postoperative facial function: H-B grading system		
		Preoperative >50/50	Postoperative >50/50	I	II	III
IC	7	3	1	7	0	0
A						
~≤10 mm	22	11	7 (64%)	16	5	1
10.1–20 mm	13	5	1 (20%)	6	3	4
20.1–30 mm	8	1[a]	1[a]	3	4	1
>30 mm	3	1	0	0	0	3
B						
~≤15 mm	31	16	8 (50%)	21	7	3
15.1–25 mm	8	0	0	1	4	3
25.1–35 mm	6	2	1[a]	3	1	2
>35 mm	1	0	0	0	0	1

IC, Intracanicular
[a] Subtotal resection

tion was evaluated more than a year after the surgery, 33 cases were categorized as HB-I, 12 cases as HB-II, and 8 cases as HB-III. Thus, 45 cases (85%) were categorized in HB-I and -II (see Table 1).

Regarding hearing preservation, measurable postoperative hearing was obtained in 22 of 48 cases. The other five cases had no measurable hearing before surgery. If we consider only those cases with preoperative hearing acuity that satisfied the so-called 50/50 rule as candidates for hearing preservation, 14 of 21 (67%) had postoperative measurable hearing. Among these 21 cases, 2 were class A, 9 were class B, 3 were class C, and 7 were class D.

Two types of classification of the intracranial portion of the tumors along with their results of functional preservation are also shown in Table 1. Regarding postoperative facial function, in both type A and type B classification, the larger the tumor becomes, the worse the postoperative facial function. However, the general tendency that the preservation rate decreases as the size of the tumor increases is seen more clearly in type B than in type A. Regarding hearing preservation, those cases with class A preoperative hearing and serviceable postoperative hearing are all found in cases that had a tumor not more than 15 mm from the porus acusticus. Thus, in analysis of our cases we could not find any reason to adopt type A classification. Although we did not perform a detailed examination of the location of the tumor within the meatus, it is difficult to obtain hearing preservation in cases where the tumor occupies the whole meatus compared with those where the tumor spares the fundus. Therefore, those cases in which the fundus of the meatus is free from tumor should be categorized separately (Fig. 1).

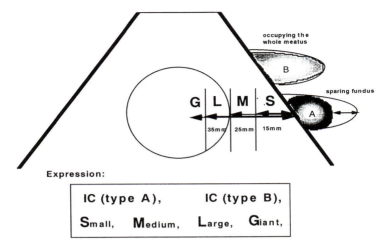

FIG. 1. Classification of acoustic neuromas by size

Discussion

Diversity of classification of tumor size of acoustic neuroma could reflect a variety of reasons related to the emphasis of this chapter. Factors that might affect the type of classification are mortality, the possibility of total removal by the surgical approach taken [2], functional preservation rate (both facial and cochlear) [3–8], treatment policy including radiotherapy [9], neurological aspect, and others. Because various classifications have been used freely so far, comparison of data from different centers has been a problem. If we are to define a certain standard classification, the following points should be taken into consideration. It should be simple, understandable, reasonable, and acceptable for those who care for patients with acoustic neuroma. Even where the criteria for the classification of acoustic neuroma have differed until now, the treatment goal for acoustic neuroma will be the same: total removal of the tumor, preservation of facial function, preservation or recovery of hearing acuity, and recovery from dysequilibrium caused by the tumor [10]. It was considered previously that sacrificing the facial nerve was a cheap price for total removal of the tumor [1]. However, no one would agree with this statement today. The anatomic preservation rate of the facial nerve has drastically improved and is now more than 90% because of recent technological developments of monitoring systems.

Although acoustic neuromas mostly arise from the vestibular nerve and not the cochlear nerve, the postoperative preservation rate of the cochlear function is still far from satisfactory. Although the detailed mechanism of hearing disorders associated with acoustic neuroma are not yet fully understood, hearing preservation or hearing recovery must surely be the priority for the future. We therefore consider it necessary that the classification method should be realistic from the point of view of functional preservation. From this aspect, type B classification may be better than type A. Those cases in which hearing was preserved in the type A classification are, as a matter of fact, those tumors of less than 15 mm from the porus as classified in type B. Although we did not have any single case of hearing preservation among patients with a tumor of 15.1–25 mm, it is generally believed that a patient with a tumor up to 25 mm could also be a candidate for hearing preservation. In addition, there is a size limitation of 25 mm for radiosurgery [11]. Accordingly, we recommend type B classification, as this would provide a reasonable success rate not only for hearing preservation but also for facial nerve function. Also, we could share the standard of other fields such as radiation therapy.

Conclusion

Based upon our experience of 53 surgical cases of acoustic neuroma and literature review, we consider the following classification of tumor size may be useful: intracanalicular tumor (type a; sparing the fundus; type b; occupying the whole meatus), small (0.1–15 mm), medium (15.1–25 mm), large (25.1–35 mm) and giant (35.1 or more).

References

1. House WF, Leutje CM, Doyle KJ (1997) Acoustic tumors: diagnosis and management, 2nd edn. Singular, San Diego
2. Haid CT, Wigand ME (1992) Advantage of the enlarged middle cranial fossa approach in acoustic neurinoma surgery. Acta Otolaryngol 112:387–407
3. Kanzaki J, Inoue Y, Kurashima K, et al. (1999) Hearing preservation in acoustic neuroma surgery: indication, preservation rate of the quality of hearing, and long term results. In: Sanna M, Taibah A, Russo A, et al. (eds) Acoustic neuroma and other CPA tumors. Monduzzi Editore, Italy, pp 615–620
4. Gardner G, Robertson JH (1988) Hearing preservation in unilateral acoustic neuroma surgery. Ann Otol Rhinol Laryngol 97:55–66
5. Moffat DA, Croxon GR, Baguley DM, et al. (1989) Facial nerve recovery after acoustic neuroma removal. J Laryngol Otol 103:169–172
6. Goel A, Sekher L, Langheinrich W, et al. (1992) Late course of preserved hearing and tinnitus after acoustic neuroma surgery. J Neurosurg 77:685–689
7. Walsh RM, Pracy JP, Gleeson MJ, et al. (1996) The value of facial nerve monitoring in acoustic tumor surgery. In: Sterkers JM, Charachon R, Sterkers O (eds) Acoustic neuroma and skull base surgery. Kugler, Amsterdam/New York, pp 127–130
8. Hinton AE, Ramsden RT, Lye RH, et al. (1992) Criteria for hearing preservation in acoustic schwannoma surgery: the concept of useful hearing. J Otolaryngol 106:500–503

9. Moller P, Myrseth E, Jensen O, et al (1996) Acoustic neuroma. Observation, surgery or gamma knife treatment. In: Sterkers JM, Charachon R, Sterkers O (eds) Acoustic neuroma and skull base surgery. Kugler, Amsterdam/New York, pp 339–341

10. Ishikawa K, Cao Z, Yasui N, et al (1999) Our result on hearing preservation in acoustic neuroma surgery by middle cranial fossa approach. Monduzzi Editore, Italy, pp 621–627

11. Harner SG (2001) Contemporary algorithm for acoustic neuroma: assessment and management. Curr Opin Otolaryngol Head Neck Surg 9:290–295

Definition of Tumor Size of Vestibular Schwannomas

Shigeaki Kobayashi, Yuichiro Tanaka, and Kazuhiro Hongo

Summary. Methods to measure the diameter of vestibular schwannomas have not been standardized in previous reports. Therefore, we undertook statistical analyses to determine the most appropriate method. Volumetry of the tumor was performed in the most recent 52 cases using magnetic resonance imaging including constructive interference in steady-state images. Pearson's correlation coefficient was determined between tumor volume and tumor diameters, including the maximum diameter of the whole tumor, maximum diameter of the cerebellopontine angle (CPA) portion, diameter through the internal auditory canal axis, $\sqrt{ab}$, and $(a + b)/2$, (where a is a diameter parallel to the petrous edge and b is a diameter perpendicular to a). The tumors were divided into three groups depending on their volume (small $<0.5\,cm^3$; medium 0.5–$2.0\,cm^3$; large $>2.0\,cm^3$); Correlation for the maxCPA was consistently strong in all three tumor groups. It was concluded that the maximum diameter of the CPA portion is the most appropriate, simplest parameter representing tumor volume.

Key words. Brain tumor, Cerebellopontine angle, Vestibular schwannoma

Introduction

Tumor size is known to be one of the most important factors for predicting functional outcome of the facial and cochlear nerves after vestibular schwannoma surgery. It is difficult to use linear measurements of the tumor diameter to represent the tumor volume correctly, however, because vestibular

Department of Neurosurgery, Shinshu University School of Medicine, 3-1-1 Asahi, Matsumoto 390-8621, Japan

schwannomas are not spherical. Various measurements [1–6] have been used in previous reports, with the result that a comparison of the surgical results from different series has been difficult.

Methods and Materials

A series of 52 patients with unilateral vestibular schwannomas was analyzed. Axially sectioned magnetic resonance images (MRI) were used for diagnosis and to measure tumor diameter. Constructive interference in steady state (CISS) imaging with a 0.6–2.6-mm slice interval was used to calculate tumor volume. The tumors were divided into three subgroups depending on the tumor volume: group I (small <0.5 cm^3), group II (medium 0.5–2.0 cm^3); and group III (large > 2 cm^3). The linear tumor diameter was measured in the axial MRI slice across the internal auditory canal (IAC). A diameter parallel to the petrous edge was designated a, and a diameter perpendicular to a was denoted b (the pons-to-petrous diameter). Five diameters were obtained for each tumor: $\sqrt{ab}$ [1]; $(a + b)/2$; maximum diameter of the cerebellopontine angle portion (maxCPA) [2,3]; maximum diameter of the whole tumor including the IAC (Max) [4,5]; and a length through the IAC axis (Axis) [6] (Fig. 1). Pearson's correlation coefficient was obtained between the tumor volume and tumor diameters for the five measuring methods.

Results

Tumor volume ranged from 0.04 to 39.2 cm^3 (mean 7.6 cm^3) in 52 tumors. There were 12 tumors in group I, 11 in group II, and 29 in group III. The maxCPA was 0–11 mm in group I, 12–18 mm in group II, and 19–57 mm in group III.

Pearson's correlation coefficients between the tumor volume and five measurements showed that Max showed the strongest correlation, followed by maxCPA, when analyzing all 52 tumors. When the comparison was restricted to group I tumors, Max and Axis showed the best correlation (Table 1).

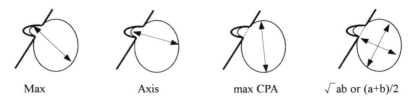

Max   Axis   max CPA $\sqrt{ab}$ or $(a+b)/2$

FIG. 1. Methods used to measure tumor diameter

TABLE 1. Correlation coefficients between tumor volume and various measurements

Tumor volume	n	Correlation coefficient, by measurement method				
		1	2	3	4	5
<0.5 cm³	12	Max	Axis	maxCPA	$(a + b)/2$	$\sqrt{ab}$
($\fallingdotseq \phi$ 1 cm)		0.923	0.923	0.828	0.815	0.809
		$P < 0.0001$	$P < 0.0001$	$P < 0.0001$	$P < 0.0001$	$P < 0.0001$
0.5–2.0 cm³	11	maxCPA	$(a + b)/2$	$\sqrt{ab}$	Axis	Max
($\fallingdotseq \phi$ 1–2 cm)		0.920	0.911	0.892	0.166	0.151
		$P < 0.0001$	$P < 0.0001$	$P < 0.0001$	NS	NS
>2.0 cm³	29	Max	maxCPA	$\sqrt{ab}$	$(a + b)/2$	Axis
($\fallingdotseq \phi$ 2 cm)		0.928	0.926	0.925	0.917	0.847
		$P < 0.0001$	$P < 0.0001$	$P < 0.0001$	$P < 0.0001$	$P < 0.0001$

For group II tumors, Max and Axis did not show significant correlation with tumor volume, whereas maxCPA, $(a + b)/2$, and $\sqrt{ab}$ showed good correlation. In group III, all five measurements attained good correlation.

Discussion

Before the MRI era the largest dimension of the tumor in the CPA was usually used because most tumors were large and the intracanalicular tumor volume had little significance. During the MRI era the IAC portion is accurately evaluated, and purely intracanalicular tumors are often encountered. Regardless of whether tumor length in the IAC is added to the tumor diameter in the CPA, it poses an important issue and various measuring methods have been adopted [1–6].

It became clear in the present study that the most appropriate measurement of the tumor diameter is not a single measurement and that it varies depending on the tumor volume. The Max or Axis parameter is recommended for small tumors (<0.5 cm³) and the maxCPA, $(a + b)/2$, or $\sqrt{ab}$ parameter for medium tumors (0.5–2.0 cm³). Any measurements can be used for large tumors (>2 cm³). It is reasonable, however, to accept maxCPA as the tumor diameter when a single measurement must be chosen while dealing with unselected tumors of various sizes.

References

1. American Academy of Otolaryngology—Head and Neck Surgery Foundation (1995) Committee on hearing and equilibrium guidelines for the evaluation of hearing preservation in acoustic neuroma (vestibular schwannoma). Otolaryngol Head Neck Surg 113: 179–180

2. Cohen NL, Lewis WS, Ransohoff J (1993) Hearing preservation in cerebellopontine angle tumor surgery: the NYU experience 1974–1991. Am J Otol 14:423–433
3. Lanman TH, Brackmann DE, Hitselberger WE (1999) Report of 190 consecutive cases of large acoustic tumors (vestibular schwannomas) removed via the translabyrinthine approach. J Neurosurg 90:617–623
4. Brackmann DE, Owens RM, Friedman RA (2000) Prognostic factors for hearing preservation in vestibular schwannoma surgery. Am J Otol 21:417–424
5. Ebersold MJ, Harner SG, Beatty CW (1992) Current results of the retrosigmoid approach to acoustic neurinoma. J Neurosurg 76:901–909
6. Dubrulle F, Ernst O, Vincent C, Vaneecloo FM, Lejeune JP, Lemaitre L (2000) Cochlear fossa enhancement at MR evaluation of vestibular schwannomas: correlation with success at hearing-preservation surgery. Radiology 215:458–462

Surgical Classification and Predictive Factors in Acoustic Neuromas

Jacques P.Y. Magnan

Summary. This study was undertaken to classify the surgical findings that lead to minimal morbidity in acoustic neuroma surgery. It is well known that hearing preservation and facial nerve function are related to tumor size. We used the Zini–Magnan classification, which is a modification of that of Tos and Thomsen and takes into account not only tumor size but also the relationship with adjacent structures. Surgical findings were recorded concerning tumor extension and relationship between cochlear nerve, facial nerve, and the acoustic neuroma, so as to define predictive factors in hearing and facial nerve preservation. From October 1993 to December 2000, 306 patients with acoustic neuroma were operated on. According to our classification, the grading was considered stage I in 37 cases (12%), stage II in 106 cases (35%), stage III in 85 cases (28%), stage IV in 75 cases (24%), and stage V in 3 cases (1%). An additional subdivision for each stage, except intracanalicular stage I, defines the aspects of the internal auditory canal: empty, a: 39 cases (13%); bottom free, b: 82 cases (27%); full filled, c: 185 cases (60%). Regardless of the level of hearing, we used the retrosigmoid approach (215 cases) for small or medium-sized tumors (stages I–III), and the translabyrinthine approach (91 cases) when the tumor was more than 2.5 cm in the cerebellopontine angle (13 cases stage III and all cases in stages IV and V). During 6 months follow-up for the 306 patients, postoperative House–Brackmann facial nerve grades were the following: grade I, 195 cases (64%); grade II, 70 cases; grade III, 18 cases; grade IV, 16 cases; grade V, 2 cases; and grade VI, 5 cases. Of 181 patients, hearing preservation was achieved in 83 cases (46%), type A in 25 cases (13.8%) and type B in 24 cases (13%). Favorable surgical factors for saving facial nerve function were facial nerve anteroinferior to the tumor and close to the cochlear nerve. Favorable surgical factors for preserving hearing were related only to easy cleavage from the tumor.

Aix-Marseille II University, ORL, Hôpital Nord, 13915 Marseille Cedex 20, France

Key words. Acoustic neuroma, Classification, Retrosigmoid, Facial, Hearing preservation

Introduction

House, Gardner, and Hugues [1] reported in 1968 that "the major principle of acoustic neuroma surgery is removal of the tumor without producing additional neurologic damage." Because it is well known that hearing preservation and facial nerve function are related to tumor size, we undertook this study to classify the surgical findings that lead to minimal morbidity in hearing and facial nerve outcomes.

Methods and Materials

Our indications were related to tumor size regardless of the preoperative hearing threshold. In intracanalicular neuromas and extended neuromas less than 2.5 cm in the cerebellopontine angle (CPA), the retrosigmoid approach was used; in neuromas 2.5 cm or greater in the CPA, the translabyrinthine approach was employed. There were some unusual cases where hearing preservation was more important for some patients, such as unilateral hearing loss or bilateral neuroma, in which a combined presigmoid and retrosigmoid approach was carried out successfully.

To grade the tumor stages and to compare results, we used the Zini–Magnan classification [2], which is a modification of that described by Tos and Thomsen [3]. Grading is based on MRI studies and intraoperative data.

Stage 1: intracanalicular tumor
Stage 2: small tumor, up to 10 mm in CPA, no contact with the brainstem
Stage 3: medium tumor, 11–25 mm, within CPA, touching and embedded in the brainstem without distortion
Stage 4: large tumor, 25–40 mm, with distortion of the brainstem and displacement of the IV ventricule
Stage 5: extralarge tumor, greater than 40 mm, extending over the middle line

For each stage we used a further classification according to intracanalicular extension:

a. Internal auditory canal (IAC): tumor process absent
b. IAC bottom free (lateral end free of tumor)
c. IAC completely filled

From October 1993 to December 2000, 306 patients with acoustic neuroma were operated on. According to our classification, the grading was considered stage I in 37 cases (12%), stage II in 106 cases (35%), stage III in 85 cases

(28%), stage IV in 75 cases (24%), and stage V in 3 cases (1%). The additional subdivision for each stage, except intracanalicular, defined the aspect of the IAC: a, 39 (13%); b, 82 (27%); c, 185 (60%).

We used the retrosigmoid approach in 215 cases for small or medium-sized tumors (stages I–III). These cases included unexpected facial nerve neuroma (3 cases) and cochlear neuroma (9 cases). The translabyrinthine approach was used in 91 cases, including 13 cases of stage III, and all cases of stages IV and V. Surgical findings were recorded concerning not only tumor extension but also the relationship between the cochlear nerve, facial nerve, and the acoustic neuroma. The course of the facial nerve in the CPA and at the meatus was variable, resulting in difficulties in determining its localization and its dissection. Regarding hearing function, three items were classified: the size of the tumor, its lateral extent in the internal auditory canal, and the ease of the cleavage between the cochlear nerve and the neuroma.

Results

Relationship Between Tumor and Facial Nerve in the Cerebellopontine Angle

The location of the facial nerve was anteroinferior to the tumor in 195 patients (64%). In this situation, the rate of postoperative facial weakness was 0.6% (1 of 145 cases) for the small and medium-sized tumors, and 26.5% (11 of 50 cases) for larger tumors. The facial nerve displaced toward the trigeminal nerve was anterosuperior to the tumor in 108 patients (35%), and the patients suffered from facial weakness in 6% (5 of 81) of cases of medium-sized tumor and in 77% of cases (21 of 27) of the larger tumors. In 2 cases, the facial nerve course was posterosuperior to the tumor process, representing an unexpected and extremely risky situation for facial function. One case was vestibular schwannoma and the other an obvious cochlear schwannoma.

Relationship Between Cochlear and Facial Nerve at the Meatus

The facial nerve was intimately close to the cochlear nerve in 180 cases, with a common arachnoid wrapping. Patients had postoperative palsy in 1 case of 137 small or medium-sized tumors and in 4 cases of 43 large-sized acoustic neuromas. The facial nerve was distant from the cochlear nerve at the level of the meatus or the cochlear nerve was not anatomically preserved with the facial nerve as the unique saved neural structure in 126 patients (40%). Patients suffered from facial weakness in 16 cases (6.5%) of 91 small and medium-sized tumors and in 30 cases (85%) of 35 large-sized tumors.

Hearing Preservation

In 181 cases, the retrosigmoid approach was used with intent to preserve hearing. Success was achieved in 83 cases (46%), including 49 patients (27%) with useful hearing, class A and B of Shelton's classification.

The predictive factors for hearing preservation in acoustic neuroma removal are the following:

1. Ease of tumor dissection from the neural structures of the acousticofacial nerve bundle was a constant surgical finding in all cases with successful hearing preservation.

2. Preoperative hearing threshold: patients with preoperative pure tone average (PTA) less than or equal to 30 db and a speech discrimination score greater than or equal to 70% had preserved hearing in 25 of 56 cases (45%). Patients with normal BAER or with otoacoustic emissions had superior hearing outcomes.

3. Hearing preservation is related to the tumor size. Nevertheless, within the group of small and medium-sized tumors we did not find significant differences between stage I and stage II for hearing preservation. In 35 intracanalicular tumors (stage I), postoperative hearing was achieved in 18 cases (51%); in 89 extracanalicular tumors (stage II), hearing preservation was achieved in 43 cases (48%). In 57 extracanalicular tumors (stage III), hearing preservation was achieved in 22 cases (38%).

4. Intracanalicular extension: when the bottom of the internal auditory canal is tumor free (stage a and b), the surgical procedure through the retrosigmoid approach is easier and faster but without any influence regarding hearing preservation in our series.

Discussion

The retrosigmoid approach is our standard procedure [4] for small and medium-sized acoustic neuroma tumors up to 2.5 cm within the CPA. The use of the retrosigmoid approach is related more to facial preservation than to hearing preservation.

The advantages of the retrosigmoid approach compared to the middle fossa approach are the following: short time of approach, easy identification of the internal auditory canal, and easy identification of tumor size and the adjacent neurovascular structures. In addition to the volume of the acoustic neuroma, a positive intraoperative prognostic factor in facial preservation is the anteroinferior localization of the facial nerve close to the cochlear nerve. In such circumstances, the dissection of the tumor can be performed en bloc from medial to lateral; the peritumoral arachnoid cleavage plane can be dissected, preserving both cochlear and facial nerves efficiently. The localization of the facial nerve course is of utmost importance as a predictive factor on facial nerve outcome when dealing with large tumors.

The lateral end of the internal auditory canal filled with tumor presents no disadvantage to the retrosigmoid approach when using an endoscopic-assisted procedure. The global result for facial nerve function preservation is 86% House–Brackmann grade I and II. In small and medium-sized tumors, facial function is preserved in 96% of cases. This finding is a major argument for surgery at an early stage of acoustic tumor growth. Furthermore, hearing function can be preserved in approximately 50% of these cases.

In all our cases with successful hearing preservation, preoperative parameters including tumor size, auditory tests, and intracanalicular extent were lesser predictive factors than the intraoperative finding of the ease of tumor excision. A clear and easy cleavage of the tumor from the adjacent neural structures, in fact, represents the most basic yet unpredictable requirement for successful hearing preservation.

Conclusion

Classification and statistical analysis of the outcomes of 306 patients with acoustic neuroma in the present study supports the use of the retrosigmoid approach for small and medium-sized tumors. The translabyrinthine approach is performed for large tumors. In addition to tumor size, several types of surgical data influence facial and hearing outcome. Favorable surgical factors for saving facial nerve function were the facial nerve anteroinferior to the tumor and closeness to the cochlear nerve. Favorable surgical factors for preserving hearing were related only to the ease of cleavage of small or medium-sized tumors from adjacent tissues.

References

1. House W, Gardner G, Hugues G (1983) Acoustic neuroma management. Am J Otol 5:87–108
2. Zini C, Magnan J, Piazza F, et al (2000) New surgical classification of acoustic neuromas. In: Sanna M (ed) Acoustic neuroma and other CPA tumors. Monduzzi, Rome, pp 117–120
3. Tos M, Thomsen J (1992) Synopsis on disagreements in measuring tumor size at the Copenhagen Acoustic Neuroma Conference. In: Acoustic neuroma. Kugler, Amsterdam, pp 975–978
4. Bruzzo M, Broder L, Chays A, et al (2000) Nos résultats actuels de la chirurgie du neurinome de l'acoustique. Ann Otolaryngol (Paris) 117:110–117

A Classification System for Vestibular Schwannomas

Tetsuji Sekiya and Shigeharu Suzuki

Summary. A classification system for vestibular schwannomas (VSs) is proposed, whereby VSs are classified first by location, and then by extent. This system is proposed because traditional classifications of VSs do not comprehensively describe lesions that grow in different patterns after arising in regions as diverse as the cerebellopontine (CP) angle, the internal auditory canal, and the region lateral to the fundus of the internal auditory canal (labyrinth). The proposed system provides surgeons information helpful in choosing the surgical approach, in estimating the difficulty of tumor excision, and in determining whether hearing might be preserved. The system also avoids confusion and misunderstanding in discussion of treatment results because it reflects the diverse biological characteristics of VSs.

Key words. Classification, Hearing, Vestibular schwannoma

Introduction

Vestibular schwannomas (VSs) have been traditionally classified according to the size of the tumor [1]. However, such classification systems do not comprehensively describe either the diverse areas in which VSs arise, or their growth patterns. We propose here a classification system for VSs that allows surgeons to envisage anatomic relationships between the tumor and surrounding structures.

Our classification system of vestibular schwannomas (Fig. 1):

Department of Neurosurgery, Hirosaki University School of Medicine, 5 Zaifu-cho, Hirosaki 036-8216, Japan

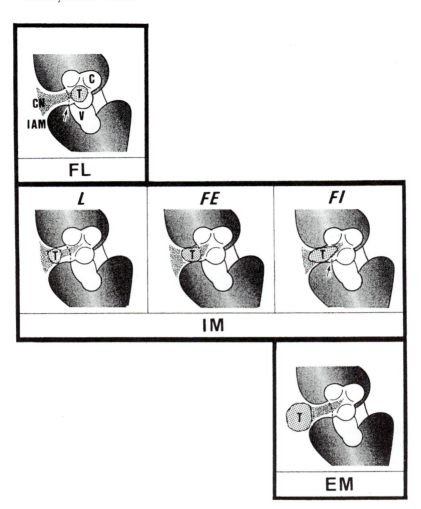

FIG. 1. Classification of vestibular schwannomas. Tumor may occupy the region lateral to the fundus of the internal auditory canal (IAC) (*arrow*), (far-lateral tumor, *FL*). Intrameatal tumor may be localized, without occupying any part of the fundus of the internal auditory canal (intrameatal-localized, *IM-L*). Intrameatal tumor extends to the fundus of the IAC but does not cross the fundus into the labyrinth (intrameatal-fundus extension, *IM-FE*). Tumor crosses the fundus to invade the labyrinth (intrameatal-fundus invasion, *IM-FI*). *C*, cochlea; *CN* cochlear nerve; *EM*, extrameatal tumor; *IAM*, external auditory meatus; *T*, tumor; *V*, vestibule

1. Far-lateral region. A few reports have indicated that VS occur in the region lateral to the fundus of the internal auditory canal, namely, the labyrinth. Far-lateral tumors (FL) may occupy the cochlea, semicircular canals, and vestibule.

2. Intrameatal region. Our experimental work indicates that the cochlear nerve and the internal auditory artery may be avulsed at the fundus of the internal auditory canal (IAC) during surgery [2,3]. The success of hearing preservation depends not only on the size of the tumor but also on the extent to which the fundus of the IAC is involved. First, the intrameatal tumor may be localized, without occupying any part of the fundus of the IAC, labeled IM-L (intrameatal-localized). The second type of intrameatal tumor extends to the fundus of the IAC but does not cross the fundus into the labyrinth, labeled IM-FE (intrameatal-fundus extension). The third type of tumor crosses the fundus to invade the labyrinth, labeled IM-FI (intrameatal-fundus invasion).

3. Region of the cerebellopontine (CP) angle cistern. Tumors in the CP angle are classified as extrameatal (EM) with an additional designation for size if needed.

Discussion

Magnetic resonance (MR) imaging has made it possible for far-lateral tumors to be diagnosed preoperatively [4–6]. The operative indication for such small tumors is controversial. At the present time, we think it most appropriate to carefully observe their growth rate and pattern with yearly MR examination. There are reports of schwannomas growing in the middle ear cavity without an IAC or CP angle component. These tumors might have originated in the far-lateral region and then grown unimpeded through the lumen of the inner ear and subsequently prolapsed through the round window into the middle ear cavity [7–9]. The technical difficulty of tumor removal depends not only upon tumor size per se but also upon the anatomic structures involved by the lesion. Our classification system is based on the biological growth pattern of VS. Most VSs originate from the IAC portion of the vestibular nerve and tend to grow mainly medially along the path of least resistance from the IAC into the CP angle. Their lateral growth is impeded by the fundus of the IAC. From the standpoint of surgery, whether a tumor is IM-FI (intrameatal-fundus invasion) is a critical issue because tumor tissue beyond the fundus may not be easily removed by the ordinary posterior fossa approach, with a possibility of subsequent tumor recurrence. Classifying tumor tissue within the IAC as only either filling or not filling the canal, therefore, is not an adequate classification system for clinical purposes. Using our classification system, confusion and misunderstanding in discussion of results of treatment of VSs may

EM-15 + IM-FE

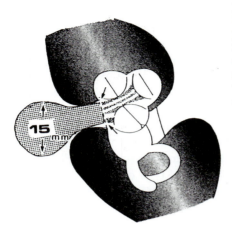

FIG. 2. This tumor is designated as EM-15 + IM-FE, because the extrameatal cerebellopontine (CP) angle portion of the tumor is 15 mm and the tumor has an intrameatal portion that extends to the fundus of the internal auditory canal. *C*, cochlea; *CN*, cochlear nerve; *IAM*, internal auditory meatus; *T*, tumor; *V*, vestibule. *Arrows*, position of the fundus of the internal auditory canal

be avoided because it reflects the diverse biological characteristics of VSs (Fig. 2).

References

1. Tos M, Thomsen J (1992) Synopsis on disagreements in measuring tumour size at the Copenhagen acoustic neuroma conference. In: Tos M, Thomsen J (eds) Acoustic neuroma. Proceedings of the first international conference on acoustic neuroma. Kugler, Amsterdam, pp 975–978
2. Sekiya T, Møller AR (1987) Avulsion rupture of the internal auditory artery during the cerebellopontine angle: a study in monkeys. Neurosurgery 21:631–637
3. Sekiya T, Møller AR (1988) Effects of cerebellar retraction on the cochlear nerve: an experimental study on rhesus monkeys. Acta Neurochir (Wien) 90:45–52
4. Donnelly MJ, Daly CA, Briggs RJS (1994) MR imaging features of an intracochlear acoustic schwannoma. J Laryngol Otol 108:1111–1114
5. Mafee MF, Lachenauer CS, Kumar A, et al (1990) CT and MR imaging of intra-labyrinthine schwannoma: report of two cases and review of the literature. Radiology 174:395–400
6. Saeed SR, Birzgalis AR, Ramsden RT (1994) Intralabyrinthine schwannoma shown by magnetic resonance imaging. Neuroradiology 36:63–64
7. Amolis CP, Lanser MJ, Jackler RK (1992) Acoustic neuroma as a middle ear mass. Otolaryngol Head Neck Surg 107:478–482
8. Stoney PJ, Rutka J, Dolan E, et al (1991) Acoustic neuroma presenting as a middle ear mass. J Otolaryngol 20:141–143
9. Woolford TJ, Birzgalis AR, Ramsden RT (1994) An extensive vestibular schwannoma with both intracranial spread and lateral extension to the external auditory canal. J Laryngol Otol 108:149–151

Measurement of Tumor Volume in Acoustic Neurinomas

Stephan R. Wolf[1], Florian Triebswetter[2], and Malte E. Wigand[2]

Summary. The so-called wait-and-scan policy was proposed in acoustic neurinoma (AN) patients with small tumors several years ago. A major effort was undertaken to classify spontaneous tumor progression as found in follow-up magnetic resonance imaging (MRI) scans. Although tumors progress in three dimensions, most authors rely exclusively on single linear measurements. Volumetric estimations from MRI data are possible but are not routinely performed by radiologists. Therefore, a calculation of tumor volume based on measurements in three axes and calculation of a sphere was adopted, and results were compared to intraoperative volume measurements of removed tumor tissue in 61 middle fossa AN cases. Intraoperative and calculated volumes were correlated ($r^2 = 0.85$). The volume model was found to be especially appropriate for medium-sized tumors. In purely intrameatal tumors, the calculated volume tended to underscore, and in larger ones to overscore, the intraoperative measurements. Although neither progress of symptoms nor intraoperative findings and outcome are well correlated to radiological findings, follow-up of tumor volume is generally proposed. Tumor volume calculated from three axes is helpful if a voxel count is not available.

Key words. Acoustic neurinoma (vestibular schwannoma), Volume measurement, intraoperative measurements, imaging, Growth studies

[1] Department of ORL, University Regensburg, HNO-Klinik, Franz-Josef-Strauss-Allee 11, D-93053, Regensburg, Germany
[2] Department of ORL, University Erlangen-Nuernberg, Erlangen, Germany

Introduction

How to measure the size of an acoustic neurinoma (AN)? This question has introduced controversies and is not yet satisfactorily answered.

In many radiological studies, one [1] or two diameters [2] of the tumor are described. Several differing measurements have been proposed, e.g., the largest diameter in the cerebellopontine angle, or the longitudinal diameter in the axis of the internal auditory canal with or without measuring the largest perpendicular diameter. However, tumors grow in three dimensions and, as in the human body where the height of a person does not reflect their weight, a simple longitudinal measurement is not well correlated to the mass of a tumor. Exact knowledge of tumor size is mandatory for a wait-and-scan policy, follow-up after radiotherapy, or for patients with residual tumor. There is general consensus that the most appropriate method would be volume estimation by voxel count, but this is not routinely available. Calculation derived from imaging is challenging if carried out on the basis of plain film material.

Material and Methods

In a consecutive series of 61 patients undergoing AN removal by the enlarged middle cranial fossa approach [3], the size of the tumor in magnetic resonance imaging (MRI) (T1 with Gd enhancement) was studied and compared to intraoperative volume measurement. Three tumor diameters were gained from MRI studies: first, in horizontal cuts in the axis of the tumor following the internal auditory canal; second, perpendicular to this axis in the largest extent; and third, in coronal sections, the largest height of the tumor in the craniocaudal direction. Volume of the tumor was calculated according to the mathematical formula of a sphere. The radius of the sphere was found by arithmetic averaging of the three diameters. A more sophisticated volume model was not applied because the intent was to provide an easy method.

Intraoperative measurement was carried out following microsurgical resection of the tumor by the enlarged middle cranial fossa approach. Tumor pieces were collected, stored in Ringer's solution, and, at the end of surgery after removing extra fluid by laying the tumor pieces on cotten, transferred to a sterile calibrated vessel (total volume, 10 ml; calibration, 0.1 ml) filled with 2 ml Ringer's solution. The effect of volume displacement by the tumor pieces was noted and the tumor prepared for histological studies.

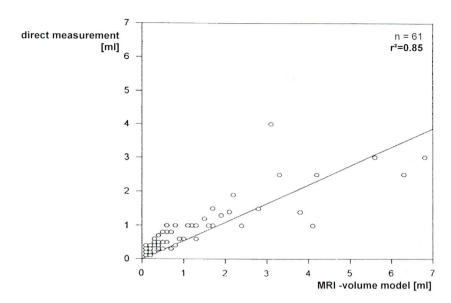

FIG. 1. Size of acoustic neurinomas. Comparison of calculation from a sphere model with three axial measurements from magnetrc resonance imaging (MRI) and direct intraoperative measurements during removal by the enlarged middle fossa approach (volume displacement; $n = 61$, small and medium-sized tumors; $r^2 = 0.85$)

Results

Tumors were classified according to Wigand's scheme in three stages: purely intracanalicular tumors (size A; $n = 13$), intra- and extracanalicular tumors without contact with the brainstem (size B; $n = 27$), and tumors with broad contact with the brainstem (size C; $n = 21$). The calculated volume was found within a range of 0.1–6.8 cm^3. Intraoperatively, volume ranged from 0.1 to 4.3 cm^3; the correlation coefficient was 0.85 (Fig. 1). Comparing different stages, the mathematical model was found to be most appropriate in patients with tumor size B, whereas intracanalicular tumors were underestimated and larger ones were found to be slightly overestimated (Fig. 1).

Discussion

Intraoperative volume measurements in patients with acoustic neurinomas (AN), to our knowledge, have not been published previously. We describe a simple method of measuring volume displacement by tumor particles. Several factors may influence the measurement: reading of the calibrated vessel is dependent on the training of the personnel, contamination with nontumor particles or with irrigation fluid is easily possible, and the surgical nurses had been advised. Surgical technique itself also has a significant influence. Tumor removal with the ultrasound scalpel is not possible because suctioning of tumor particles will cause loss of tumor fragments. HF coagulation, rarely used in our hands, and other methods of tumor reduction may also influence the result. Nevertheless, intraoperative volume measurement is easily possible with minimal effort. In small and medium-sized tumors, the correlation to preoperative calculation based on a spherical model is sufficient. Further adaptation to different volume models [4] might additionally improve the results in large tumors but would provide less acceptance. The calculation shown herein can be proposed for tumors of the internal auditory meatus and the cerebellopontine angle of less than 15 mm extrameatal expansion.

The most accurate procedure would be the exact volumetric calculation derived from voxels [5–7], preferably in noncontrast-enhanced sequences (e.g., constructive interference in steady state CISS). In Germany, only a few radiologists are able to supply these data. Images are still performed by several protocols, with different geometry. Recalculating voxels is vague, time consuming, and cannot be applied in all patients. Semiautomatic systems have been described [8] but are not yet established. Calculation based on measurements in three axes is easy and offers an estimation of tumor volume. It may be especially helpful if different radiological institutions have performed the follow-up images. However, tumor volume and function loss are not correlated. Small tumors even in a nongrowth period may cause progressive symptoms, and large, growth-active tumors may not lead to increasing functional problems. Only the neurotologist is able to supervise the situation of the patient—symptoms, tumor size, and further development. Volume calculation derived from MRI studies could be helpful in one aspect of AN development. So long as tumor volume is not measured from voxel counts on a routine basis, a three-dimensional sphere model can be helpful.

References

1. Sakamoto T, Fukuda S, Inuyama Y (2001) Hearing loss and growth rate of acoustic neuromas in follow-up observation period. Auris Nasus Larynx 28:223–227
2. Ogawa K, Kanzaki J, Ogawa S, et al (1991) The growth rate of acoustic neuromas. Acta Otolaryngol (Stockh) (Suppl) 487:157–163
3. Wigand ME, Haid CT, Berg M, et al (1982) The enlarged transtemporal approach to the cerebellopontine angle; technique and indications. Acta Otorhinolaryngol (Ital) 2:571–583
4. Somville J, De Beuckeleer L, De Schepper A, et al (2001) Reliability of measuring volume by different methods for tumors of the musculoskeletal system. Acta Orthop Belg 67: 338–343

5. Fiirgaard B, Pedersen CB, Lundorf E (1997) The size of acoustic neuromas: CT and MRI. Neuroradiology 39:599–601
6. Laasonen EM, Troup H (1986) Volume growth rate of acoustic neurinomas. Neuroradiology 28:203–207
7. Long SA, Arriaga M, Nelson RA (1993) Acoustic neuroma volume: MRI-based calculations and clinical implications. Laryngoscope 103:1093–1096
8. Sarazin L, Jolivet O, Doyon D (1993) Computerized evaluation of tumor volume with MRI. Applications to the surveillance of acoustic neurinoma. J Radiol 74:455–460

Tumor Volume Measurements of Acoustic Neuromas with MR Imaging

Ichiro Yamada[1], Atsushi Komatsuzaki[2], Atsunobu Tsunoda[2], and Yoshihiro Noguchi[2]

Summary. Although clinical decisions are based on the measurement of diameter, tumor volume is a more clinically relevant parameter in the management of patients with acoustic neuromas. On the basis of the voxel-count method and three-dimensional (3D) constructive interference in steady state (CISS) MR imaging, we evaluated ellipsoid formulas in conventional spin-echo (SE) magnetic resonance (MR) imaging in tumor volume measurements of acoustic neuromas. Twenty-two patients with acoustic neuromas were examined using high-resolution 3D-CISS and SE imaging with a 1.5-T system. Tumor volume determined by SE imaging with ellipsoid formulas was over-estimated when compared with volumes obtained by 3D-CISS with the voxel-count method (the standard reference method). However, tumor volume obtained using SE imaging with ellipsoid formulas showed a high correlation with volumes determined by the reference standard ($P < 0.0001$). The use of regression equations allowed a more accurate evaluation of the tumor volume determined on the basis of tumor diameters observed in SE images. Thus, we recommend the use of regression equations for more accurate evaluation of the tumor volume of acoustic neuromas when determined on the basis of tumor diameters.

Key words. Volume measurement, Acoustic neuroma, MR imaging, High resolution, CISS

[1] Department of Radiology, Faculty of Medicine, [2] Department of Otorhinolaryngology, Tokyo Medical and Dental University, 1-5-45 Yushima, Bunkyo-ku, Tokyo 113–8519, Japan

Introduction

Although clinical decisions are based on the measurement of diameter, tumor volume is a more clinically relevant parameter in the management of patients with acoustic neuromas [1,2]. Recently, high-resolution three-dimensional (3D) MR imaging using the constructive interference in steady state (CISS) sequence has come to be employed for evaluating acoustic neuromas [3,4] because it allows a much more detailed study than does conventional spin-echo (SE) imaging [5,6]. In this study, we evaluated the use of ellipsoid formulas in SE imaging in tumor volume measurements of acoustic neuromas by comparison with the voxel-count method with 3D-CISS imaging [7].

Materials and Methods

Patients

The subjects studied were 22 patients with acoustic neuromas who underwent magnetic resonance (MR) imaging in the past 2 years. In these 22 consecutive cases, acoustic neuromas were suspected after MR imaging. Eleven of the 22 patients were men and 11 were women; their ages ranged from 30 to 78 years (mean, 52 years). All patients underwent surgery, and all tumors were histopathologically confirmed as neuromas.

Imaging Examinations

A 1.5-T superconducting system with a 25 mT/m maximum gradient capability (Magnetom Vision; Siemens, Erlangen, Germany), and a circularly polarized head coil was used to obtain all MR images. High-resolution 3D MR imaging was performed using a 3D-CISS sequence with the following parameters: 12.3/5.9 (repetition time ms/echo time ms), a flip angle of 70°, and one signal acquired. The acquisition matrix was 384×512 for a field of view of 165×220 mm. The other imaging parameters included a slab thickness of 32 mm and 46 slices, which gave a slice thickness of 0.7 mm and a voxel size of 0.1 mm^3.

Axial T1-weighted SE (450/14) and T2-weighted turbo SE (3500/96; echo train length, 7) MR images were obtained, with 2 signals acquired. After an intravenous administration of 0.1 mmol/kg of gadopentetate dimeglumine (Mangevist; Schering, Osaka, Japan), axial and coronal T1-weighted SE (450/14) images were obtained. All these images were obtained with a field of view of 165×220 mm, a matrix of 192×256, and a slice thickness of 3 mm without an interslice gap.

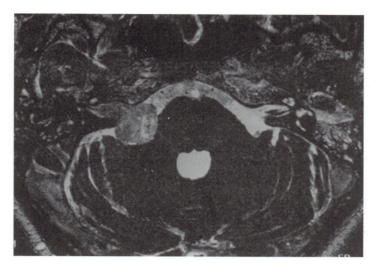

Fɪɢ. 1. Axial three-dimensional constructive interference in steady state (3D-CISS) image (12.3/5.9; flip angle, 70°) in a 38-year-old man with acoustic neuroma shows a well-defined, extraaxial mass lesion in the right cerebellopontine angle cistern and internal auditory canal. The tumor volume for the total tumor and the extrameatal tumor was calculated with the voxel-count method. (From [7], with permission)

Image Analysis

In 3D-CISS imaging, the tumor volume for the total tumor and the extrameatal tumor was calculated with the voxel-count method at a workstation (Fig. 1). The tumor was segmented by manually tracing the boundaries of the tumor on each slice. The tumor volume was then calculated automatically by adding all voxel volumes lying within the boundaries of the tumor. The mean of the four voxel-count measurements was then used as the standard reference tumor volume.

In SE imaging, the tumor volume for the total tumor and the extrameatal tumor was calculated by using the ellipsoid formula: volume $= abc \times \pi/6$. Furthermore, we used the following four approximation formulas: $(ab)^{3/2} \times \pi/6$; $[(a + b)/2]^3 \times \pi/6$; $a^3 \times \pi/6$; and $b^3 \times \pi/6$. The following three orthogonal diameters for the total tumor and the extrameatal tumor were measured: a, maximum diameter (mm) along the pyramid; b, maximum diameter (mm) perpendicular to the pyramid; and c, maximum height (mm). The diameters were measured on axial and coronal contrast-enhanced T1-weighted SE images. The mean of the four ellipsoid formula measurements was used to calculate the accuracy.

Statistical Analysis

The accuracy of the tumor volume measurements obtained with the ellipsoid formulas and SE imaging was investigated by calculating the difference between the volume obtained using the ellipsoid formulas and that obtained by 3D-CISS imaging with the voxel-count method (the standard reference method). Linear regression analysis was performed to equate the tumor volume obtained with the ellipsoid formulas and SE imaging with that obtained with the voxel-count method with 3D-CISS imaging. *P* values of less than 0.05 were considered to be significant.

Results

Tumor Volume Measurements

The mean volumes of 22 acoustic neuromas are shown in Table 1. In Figs. 2 and 3, the tumor volumes obtained by using the ellipsoid formula with SE imaging are compared with those obtained by using the voxel-count method with 3D-CISS imaging (the standard reference method). The total tumor volumes obtained using SE imaging with the ellipsoid formula were significantly larger (mean difference, $692\,mm^3$; relative difference, 35%) than those obtained via 3D-CISS imaging ($P < 0.01$). The extrameatal tumor volumes obtained with the ellipsoid formula and SE imaging were also larger (mean difference, $155\,mm^3$; mean relative difference, 5%) than those obtained with the standard reference method, although this difference was not significant. Thus, compared with the standard reference tumor volumes, calculation of tumor volumes by applying the ellipsoid formula to SE imaging resulted in substantial overestimation of acoustic neuroma volumes.

In the case of other approximation formulas, calculation of tumor volumes by applying the formulas to SE imaging also resulted in overestimation of acoustic neuroma volumes compared with the standard reference tumor volumes (see Table 1). However, in the case of volume = $b^3 \times \pi/6$, the extrameatal tumor volume was underestimated.

Correlations of Tumor Volume Measurements

The tumor volumes for the total tumor and extrameatal tumor obtained by SE imaging with the ellipsoid formula showed a high correlation with the standard reference tumor volumes measured using 3D-CISS imaging ($P < 0.0001$ for both) (Figs. 2,3). The ellipsoid-based measurements using SE imaging had a systemic overestimation in tumor volume measurements. The total tumor volume could be estimated by using the following equation ($P < 0.0001$): total tumor volume = $-26.407 + 0.740 \times abc\ \pi/6$. The extrameatal tumor volume could be estimated by using the following equation ($P <$

TABLE 1. Comparison of tumor volume measurements of acoustic neuromas: ellipsoid formulas with spin-echo (SE) imaging versus the voxel-count method with 3D-CISS imaging

Calculation method	Mean	SD	P value
Total tumor volume			
Voxel count with 3D-CISS	1865	2242	NA
abc × π/6	2557	2969	<0.01
$(ab)^{3/2}$ × π/6	3035	3274	<0.001
$[(a + b)/2]^3$ × π/6	3102	3280	<0.001
a^3 × π/6	2606	3521	<0.05
b^3 × π/6	3869	3382	<0.0001
Extrameatal tumor volume			
Voxel count with 3D-CISS	1621	2231	NA
abc × π/6	1776	2561	NS
$(ab)^{3/2}$ × π/6	1752	2671	NS
$[(a + b)/2]^3$ × π/6	1804	2703	NS
a^3 × π/6	2606	3521	<0.01
b^3 × π/6	1213	2044	<0.0001

All measurements are in cubic millimeters
3D-CISS, three-dimensional constructive interference in steady state; NA, not available; NS, not significant

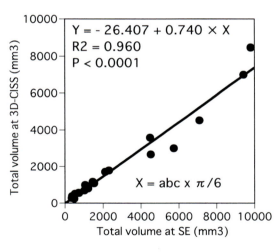

FIG. 2. Relations between total tumor volumes measured by spin-echo (SE) imaging and those measured by 3D-CISS imaging in 22 acoustic neuromas. Plot of the total tumor volume measured by SE imaging versus that measured by 3D-CISS imaging shows a significant correlation ($r = 0.980$, $P < 0.0001$). (From [7], with permission)

$Y = -26.407 + 0.740 \times X$
$R2 = 0.960$
$P < 0.0001$

$X = abc \times π/6$

0.0001): extrameatal tumor volume = 81.729 + 0.867 × abc π/6. Therefore, the tumor volume of acoustic neuromas could be assessed by using the following equations: Total tumor volume = −26.407 + 0.387 × abc; and extrameatal tumor volume = 81.729 + 0.454 × abc.

    In the case of other approximation formulas, also, the tumor volumes for the total tumor and extrameatal tumor obtained by SE imaging with the

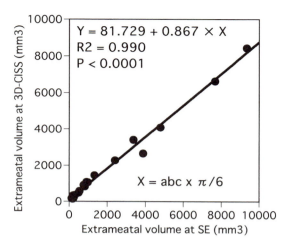

FIG. 3. Relations between extra-meatal tumor volumes measured by SE imaging and those measured by 3D-CISS imaging in 22 acoustic neuromas. Plot of the extrameatal tumor volume measured by SE imaging versus that measured by 3D-CISS imaging shows a significant correlation ($r = 0.995$, $P < 0.0001$). (From [7], with permission)

formulas showed a high correlation with tumor volumes obtained using the standard reference method.

Discussion

Our data demonstrate that tumor volume calculations obtained by using SE imaging with ellipsoid formulas resulted in substantial, systematic overestimation of the tumor volume compared with those obtained by using 3D-CISS imaging with the voxel-count method (the standard reference method). The inaccuracy occurs because the acoustic neuroma is not a true ellipsoid.

High-resolution 3D-CISS MR imaging has been used for evaluating acoustic neuromas [3,4]. 3D-CISS imaging incorporates a high spatial resolution (0.4×0.4 mm), thin slices (0.7 mm), and a small voxel size (0.1 mm³), and this allows a much more detailed and accurate examination of acoustic neuromas than does conventional SE imaging [5,6]. Therefore, we believe that tumor volumes assessed at high-resolution 3D-CISS imaging with the voxel-count method can be used as the standard reference method for volume measurement of acoustic neuromas. In contrast, the inaccuracy of the tumor volume calculations using SE imaging with ellipsoid formulas, found in this study, was probably owing to a lower spatial resolution and thicker slices in SE imaging and inappropriate approximation to an ellipsoid.

However, tumor volumes determined by SE imaging with the ellipsoid formula showed a high correlation with the tumor volumes determined by 3D-CISS imaging ($P < 0.0001$). The ellipsoid-based measurements with SE imaging had a systemic overestimation in tumor volume measurements. Therefore, the tumor volume could be estimated by using the following equations ($P < 0.0001$): total tumor volume = $-26.407 + 0.387 \times abc$; and extrameatal tumor volume = $81.729 + 0.454 \times abc$. These equations would allow more accurate evaluation of the tumor volume of acoustic neuromas based on tumor diameters measured by SE imaging.

The method to measure the diameter of acoustic neuromas has not been established. Our present results suggest that any diameter of the tumor tends to overestimate the tumor volume when the volume is calculated from ellipsoid formulas. We recommend using regression equations for more accurate evaluation of the tumor volume of acoustic neuromas when calculated on the basis of tumor diameters.

In conclusion, tumor volume measurement by SE imaging with ellipsoid formulas was overestimated when compared with that measured using 3D-CISS and the voxel-count method (the reference standard method). However, tumor volume obtained using SE imaging showed a high correlation with that obtained using the reference standard. The regression equation allowed more accurate evaluation of tumor volume when calculated on the basis of tumor diameters measured by SE imaging. We recommend using regression equations for more accurate evaluation of tumor volume of acoustic neuromas when measured on the basis of tumor diameters.

References

1. Long SA, Arriaga M, Nelson RA (1993) Acoustic neuroma volume: MRI-based calculations and clinical implications. Laryngoscope 103:1093–1096
2. Fiirgaard B, Pedersen CB, Lundorf E (1997) The size of acoustic neuromas: CT and MRI. Neuroradiology 39:599–601
3. Stuckey SL, Harris AJ, Mannolini SM (1996) Detection of acoustic schwannoma: use of constructive interference in the steady state three-dimensional MR. Am J Neuroradiol 17:1219–1225
4. Hermans R, Van der Goten A, De Foer B, et al (1997) MRI screening for acoustic neuroma without gadolinium: value of 3DFT-CISS sequence. Neuroradiology 39: 593–598
5. Casselman JW, Kuhweide R, Deimling M, et al (1993) Constructive interference in steady-state 3DFT MR imaging of the inner ear and cerebellopontine angle. Am J Neuroradiol 14:47–57
6. Stillman AE, Remley K, Loes DJ, et al (1994) Steady-state free precession imaging of the inner ear. Am J Neuroradiol 15:348–350
7. Yamada I, Tsunoda A, Noguchi Y, et al (2000) Tumor volume measurements of acoustic neuromas with three-dimensional constructive interference in steady state and conventional spin-echo MR imaging. J Magn Reson Imaging 12:826–832

Volume Analysis and Examination of Parameters of the Tumor Diameter by Three-dimensional Reconstruction of Vestibular Schwannomas

Toshiyuki Tanaka[1], Kaori Hara[1], Yumiko Hata[1], and Takanobu Kunihiro[2]

Summary. Otolaryngologists diagnose the ingravescence of vestibular schwannoma (acoustic neuroma) by the pathology in the internal auditory meatus based on magnetic resonance imaging (MRI) and computed tomography (CT) images. The tumor diameter parameter is necessary for distinguishing the ingravescence of the tumor from the value of the parameter and for determining medical care. The methods used for measuring and computing the diameters of vestibular schwannomas differ among doctors. An international definition has not yet been established regarding the tumor diameters parameter of vestibular schwannomas. In this study we computed tumor volumes based on the tumor area determined from MRI images. We were able to determine visually and numerically the shape of tumors from the three-dimensional reconstruction of the lesions using MRI images. It has been shown by many computations and comparisons that our proposed indices were better than the widely used previous parameters.

Key words. Volume analysis, Three-dimensional reconstruction, Tumor diameter, Vestibular schwannoma

Introduction

Otolaryngologists diagnose the ingravescence of vestibular schwannomas (acoustic neuromas) by the pathology in the internal auditory meatus based on magnetic resonance imaging (MRI) and computed tomography (CT)

[1] Department of Applied Physics and Physico-Informatics, Faculty of Science and Technology, Keio University, 3-14-1 Hiyoshi, Kohoku-ku, Yokohama 223-8522, Japan
[2] Department of Otorhinolaryngology, School of Medicine, Keio University, 35 Shinanomachi, Shinjuku-ku, Tokyo 160-8582, Japan

images. The tumor diameter parameter is necessary for distinguishing the ingravescence of the tumor from the value of the parameter and for determining medical care. The methods used for measuring and computing the diameters of vestibular schwannomas differ among doctors. At present, 11 tumor parameters are used around the world. The main parameters are $\sqrt{a \times b}, a + b,$ and $(a + b)/2,$ where a is the length of the long axis of the tumor and b is the length of the short axis. Methods for measuring the shape of the parameters also differ. An international definition has not yet been established for the tumor diameter parameter of vestibular schwannomas.

In this study a shape extraction method was developed using image processing. Computation of volumes and three-dimensional (3D) reconstruction of tumors were carried out based on the obtained shape of tumors. We propose new indices for the shape parameter and compare those indices with the parameters used around the world.

Method

Data Used for this Research

We used contrast T1-weighted MRI images. The thickness of the MRI slices was 2mm. These were 28 images obtained for each case, and they were 256×256 pixels, with 24-bit BMP format and gray scale with 256 tones. These images were used for clinical diagnosis.

Tumor Classification

Tumors were classified as general-type tumors depending on the site of the tumor, those in the internal meatus (IM), and cystic-type tumors: type I (general), type II (IM), and type III (cystic), respectively. These tumor types are shown in Fig. 1. A vestibular schwannoma (acoustic neuroma) is encircled in each part of Fig. 1. An abscess sometimes becomes apparent with general tumors, as shown in Fig. 1a.

Computation of Volume

Extraction of Tumor from MRI Images

For images that have tones that are markedly different from those of others, binarization was carried out on the original images, and the shapes of the tumors were determined. The threshold of binarization was based on our experience. When the binarization could not be carried out on the original images because of little difference in image tones, contour lines were interpolated and emphasized by the spline function. After emphasizing the contour lines, binarization was carried out to determine the shape of the tumors.

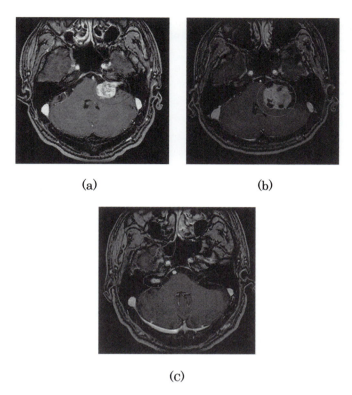

(a)   (b)

(c)

FIG. 1a–c. Magnetic resonance imaging (MRI) images of acoustic neuroma. **a** type I (general) tumor, **b** type II (IM) tumor, and **c** type III (cystic) tumor. Tumors are *encircled*

The pixels within the tumor shape were then automatically counted by computer. The tumor volume was computed using voxels, which are the volume surrounded by pixels. Spatial data for the MRI images are necessary for volume computation. Because the number of MRI images of the tumors are different depending on the size of the tumor, we established a system whereby the number of images can be input with the computer keyboard. A slice thickness of 2 mm corresponds to 2.4 pixels, where 1 pixel corresponds to 0.833 mm from our measurements. Figure 2 shows the model for volume computation.

Computation of Parameters

Parameters were computed from the image that had the maximal area of tumor on MRI images. The parameters for five tumors were measured according to the length (Fig. 3). The previous parameters and our proposed parameters are listed in Table 1. Table 2 shows the correspondence of the tumor type with the number of parameters.

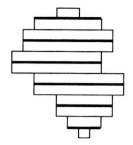

FIG. 2. Model for volume computation. Thick lines indicate the area of tumor obtained from MRI images

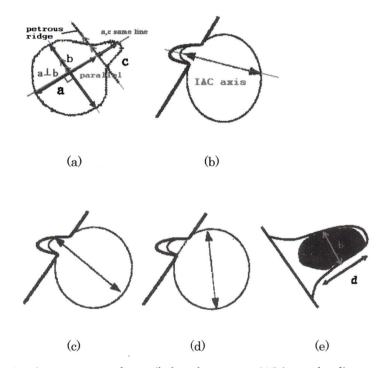

(a)

(b)

(c)

(d)

(e)

FIG. 3. Previous parameters for vestibular schwannoma. *IAC*, internal auditory canal

Three-dimensional Display of Tumors

Control points on the graphics were created by taking the points that were on the contour of the tumor at every 30° of the central angle. 3D images were prepared using those control points and OpenGL, a computer graphics library. With this system we can exchange the visual direction and the direction of lighting using the computer mouse and keyboard.

TABLE 1. Previous parameters and proposed parameters

Previous parameters

① a
② b
③ ab
④ $\sqrt{ab}$
⑤ $(a + c)/2$
⑥ $a + c$
⑦ $b(a + c)$
⑧ Max
⑨ MaxCPA
⑩ Axis
⑪ c
⑫ cd
⑬ $\sqrt{cd}$
⑭ $(c + d)/2$
⑮ $b(a + c)n$
⑯ abn
⑰ cdn

Axis, maximal length, which is parallel to the internal meatus and includes the inside of the internal meatus; Max, maximal length of the tumor including that in the meatus; MaxCPA, maximal length along all directions; n, product of the thickness of the MRI slice and number of images with tumors

TABLE 2. Tumor types and corresponding parameters

Tumor type	Corresponding parameter[a]
I: general	①–⑩, ⑮, ⑯
II: IM	⑪–⑭, ⑰
III: cystic	①–⑤, ⑧–⑩, ⑯

IM, internal meatus
[a] See Table 1

Results and Discussion

An example of 3D reconstruction is shown in Fig. 4. The computed results of the parameters and volumes are shown in Fig. 5 for a type I tumor. The horizontal axis in Fig. 5 indicates the subjects, and the vertical axis represents the normalized values for tumor diameter parameters and computed volumes. The values of all the parameters and volumes are normalized in Fig. 5 so the maximal values are unity. The parameters of the other types (types II and III) had similar results. The correlation coefficient reached 0.97463 via a com-

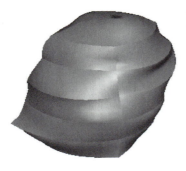

FIG. 4. Three-dimensional reconstruction of vestibular schwannoma by our method

putation based on the computed volumes and the values of the parameters. This result shows that the proposed parameter is better than the widely used previous parameters.

In this study we determined the shape of the tumor visually and numerically by 3D reconstruction from MRI images. We propose a tumor diameter parameter and constructed a diagnosis-supporting system. The shapes of acoustic neuromas were determined from MRI images, such as contrast T1-weighted head axial sections. Contour emphasis, hole-mending processing, and binarization were carried out to determine the shape of the tumor. By contour emphasis with spline function, we could extract the tumor region that had blurred contours. Our method of shape extraction was valid for most of the acoustic neuromas. The extracted shapes corresponded to the tumors in the original images. It seems that these neuroma contours were sufficient for computing the areas and 3D reconstructions.

We obtained the control points of graphics from the contour data for the tumors. Acoustic neuromas underwent 3D reconstruction using control points and the graphic library OpenGL. We stereoscopically determined almost all of the shapes of the acoustic neuromas. However, obviously, some shapes were constructed by combining small parts of the tumor. It will be necessary in the next phase to solve this problem. Graphics were rapidly carried out by displaying and rotating the tumor. Tumor shapes were determined in real time, as we could see the tumor in arbitrary directions.

Tumor volumes were computed from the area data of the tumor. The computation method was compensated so the error of the volume was small. The results of volume computation appeared valid for the diagnostic index. We compared the computed volumes with our proposed indices and previous parameters using the graphs and Pearson's correlation coefficient. As a result, the most adequate parameter was $b(a + c)n$ for the general type, *dbn* for the IM type, and *abn* for the cystic type (see Table 1, Fig. 3 for definition of parameter components). Multiplication of three components was necessary for computation of each type: the length of the tumor in the direction parallel to

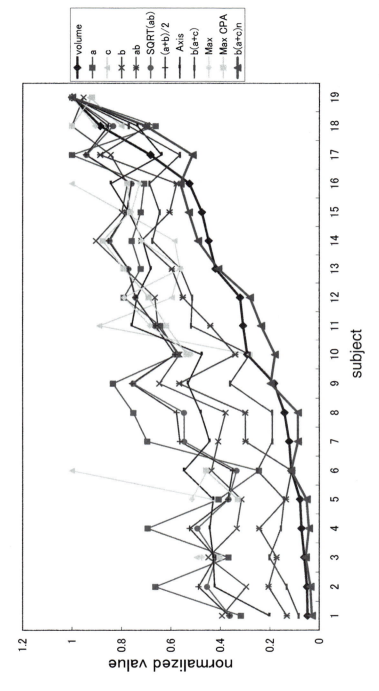

FIG. 5. Normalized values of previous parameters, our proposed parameters, and computed volumes

the internal auditory meatus; the length in the direction perpendicular to the internal auditory meatus; and the product of the number of MRI slices and their thickness. Measurements based on the internal auditory meatus were valid for the tumor diameter, as the error in the measuring step was reduced. Our proposed parameter in the vertical direction strongly correlated with the maximal length in the direction perpendicular to the vestibular schwannoma measured from the coronal image. Therefore we obtained adequate volumes only from the axial MRI image.

We propose valid tumor diameter parameters and their computational methods for vestibular schwannomas. The proposed parameter is easily measured and can be computed using only axial images (no coronal images). This method is useful for supporting the diagnosis and reducing the amount of work involved.

Conclusions

This chapter reports a diagnosis-supporting system for vestibular schwannomas using the proposed shape parameter. This parameter is based on the volume of the tumor, which was computed by 3D reconstruction from MRI images. First, we obtained the contour of the tumor from the MRI image. The obtained contours coincided well with those of the tumor in the original image. This was a good result for computing the volume from the contours of tumors. 3D reconstruction was performed using the contours obtained with the OpenGL graphics program. We could then visualize the shape of the tumor, as we could see it in arbitrary directions. Next, we computed the volume of tumor based on the contours obtained from MRI images by multiplying the area of the tumor and the slice thickness of the MRI images. It seemed that the obtained volumes were sufficiently accurate to determine the real volume. Finally, our proposed shape parameters, which corresponded to the computed volume, were better than those obtained by previous methods.

References

1. Tos M, Thomesen J (2001) Proposal for reporting size of vestibular schwannoma. Keio J Med 50(suppl 4):14
2. Kobayashi S, Tanaka Y, Hongo K (2001) Definitions of tumor size, medial type tumor and cystic tumor in vestibular schwannmas. Keio J Med 50(supple 4):21–22
3. Kanzaki J, Inoue Y, Kunihiro T (2001) Measurement of tumor size. Keio J Med 50(suppl 4):19–20
4. Reference/session I (2001) Tumor size. Keio J Med 50(suppl 4):30–36
5. NURBS (nonuniform rational B—spline) curve and surface. http://www.nakl.t.u-tokyo.ac.jp/~furu/NURBS/nurbs-jp.html.

Part 2
Facial Nerve Function

Moffat Classification of Facial Nerve Function

David A. Moffat

Summary. A reliable and sensitive facial nerve grading system is necessary to accurately assess facial nerve function after injury and to enable a meaningful comparison of facial nerve outcome after vestibular schwannoma surgery between surgical units. A number of previously published facial nerve grading systems have been proposed. The House–Brackmann (HB) grading system for facial nerve function, which was adopted as a universal standard for grading facial nerve recovery by the Facial Nerve Disorders Committee of the American Academy of Otolaryngology—Head and Neck Surgery in 1985, has moderate test–retest reliability and interobserver agreement. The deficiencies of this grading system are that HB grade III is unsatisfactory and poorly discriminatory with regard to the eye and that no account has been taken of nervus intermedius function. Also, there is no means of recording the presence of synkinesis and hemifacial spasm. This chapter proposes a new facial nerve grading system that corrects these shortcomings.

Key words. Facial nerve, Classification, Vestibular schwannoma, Grading system, Acoustic neuroma

Introduction

A reliable and sensitive facial nerve grading system is necessary to accurately assess facial nerve function after injury and to enable a meaningful comparison of facial nerve outcome after vestibular schwannoma surgery between surgical units. A number of facial nerve grading systems have been published [1–13]. House [8] published a detailed and critical analysis of these systems

Department of Otoneurological and Skull Base Surgery, Addenbrooke's Hospital, Hills Road, Cambridge University Teaching Hospitals Trust, Cambridge, CB2 2QQ, UK

in 1983 and proposed a grading system that incorporated their strengths and eradicated their weaknesses. He divided facial nerve grading systems into three categories: gross, regional, and specific.

Gross systems [1,3,5,8] give an overall grading of facial function. No effort is made to weight different areas of the face or to consider secondary effects such as synkinesis or mass movement. Regional systems [2,4,6] require that an observer assess different areas of the face independently. Facial movements in these areas are then summed and scores expressed either in nominal form or as a percentage of normal. Specific systems [7,9,10] address the presence or absence of various associated symptoms and signs, and utilize a scoring system for qualitative and quantitative defects. Secondary effects are scored separately.

Recently proposed facial grading systems have either been objective or subjective. The Burres–Fisch linear measurement index (BF-LMI), published in 1986 [11], is an objective system that involves the measurement of five standard facial expressions. In 1990, Croxon et al. [14] compared the HB facial grading system with the BF-LMI with the purpose of determining which of the two systems would be best for clinical application. The authors found a high degree of correlation between the two systems in spite of the fact that the HB scale was subjective and qualitative and the BF-LMI was objective and quantitative. It was stated that the BF-LMI was time consuming and cumbersome to use. Murty et al. in 1994 [12] proposed a simplified version of the BF-LMI, and this method has also demonstrated a high degree of correlation with the HB facial grading system using a desktop digital imaging program.

As part of an excellent overview, Chee and Nedzelski [13] proposed a subjective system entitled the Sunnybrook (Toronto) facial grading system. This subjective method assesses the face at rest and during voluntary movements. It also assesses the presence or absence of secondary defects associated with each of five voluntary movements and also grades the severity of these if present. The authors suggest the use of the HB facial grading system for stable facial nerve dysfunction but advocate the Sunnybrook system for monitoring changes in facial function because of its sensitivity and reliability.

The House–Brackmann (HB) grading system for facial nerve function was adopted as a universal standard for grading facial nerve recovery by the Facial Nerve Disorders Committee of the American Academy of Otolaryngology— Head and Neck Surgery in 1985 [10]. It has been used throughout the world since then and has enabled a meaningful comparison of facial nerve outcome after vestibular schwannoma surgery to be made between surgical units. House [8] proposed a six-point descriptive scale (Table 1) concluding that a gross system was the simplest and most practical to use clinically. In 1984, Brackmann and Barrs [9] provided an easy objective method of measuring facial function to assist in placing patients in the proper HB grade. The

TABLE 1. House–Brackmann facial nerve grading system

Grade	Description	Characteristics
I	Normal	Normal facial function in all areas

II	Mild dysfunction	Gross: slight weakness noticeable on close inspection; may have very slight synkinesis
		At rest: normal symmetry and tone
		Motion
		  Forehead: moderate to good function
		  Eye: complete closure with minimum effort
		  Mouth: slight asymmetry

III	Moderate dysfunction	Gross: obvious but not disfiguring difference between two sides; noticeable but not severe synkinesis, contracture and/or hemifacial spasm
		At rest: normal symmetry and tone
		Motion:
		  Forehead: slight to moderate movement
		  Eye: complete closure with effort
		  Mouth: slightly weak with maximum effort

IV	Moderately severe dysfunction	Gross: obvious weakness and/or disfiguring asymmetry
		At rest: normal symmetry and tone
		Motion:
		  Forehead: none
		  Eye: incomplete closure
		  Mouth: asymmetrical with maximum effort

V	Severe dysfunction	Gross: only barely perceptible motion
		At rest: asymmetry
		Motion:
		  Forehead: none
		  Eye: incomplete closure
		  Mouth: slight movement

VI	Total paralysis	No movement

movements of the eyebrow and corner of the mouth are measured and the results are compared with measurements of the unaffected side. Movements are measured using a scale with 0.25-cm divisions; there is a total possible score of 8 (4, or 1 cm for the mouth and 4, or 1 cm, for the eyebrow). These results are easily converted to the six-point scale. Various investigators have attempted to validate its reliability and sensitivity. Subjective assessments by Evans et al. [15] indicated an interobserver reliability of 93%, concluding that it was a robust system. Ross et al. [16] reported that clinical improvement could be detected in patients with facial paralysis over time even though the HB grade remained the same, casting doubt on its sensitivity as a grading tool. Rickenmann et al. [17] pointed out that when compared with a global reference the HB facial grading system did not meet the Carmines and Zeller [18] criteria required of a grading system of international standard. Correlations with objective methods have been applied since the availability of newer facial imaging technology [19]. Ahrens et al. [20] used a computer-assisted rapid grading system and with computer-performed scoring found a moderate test–retest reliability and interobserver agreement.

The well-recognized problem with this classification, however, has been House grade III. The attainment of this grade of function has generally been regarded by surgeons as a satisfactory outcome and indeed most series quote House grades I–III as satisfactory and House IV–VI as unsatisfactory. Many patients with this grade of facial nerve function are, however, incapacitated with a dry eye, or exposure keratitis, and many require a lateral or medial tarsorrhaphy or a gold weight in the upper eyelid.

The HB facial grading system does not take into account nervus intermedius function. The results of facial nerve outcome following vestibular schwannoma surgery have ignored the sensory component of the nerve [21].

In view of the effect of aberrant regeneration of the facial nerve on the patient's quality of life [22] with respect to nervus intermedius and the possible sequelae of crocodile tears, metallic taste in the mouth or dysgeusia, dry eye, and exposure keratitis, it is important to record the results with regard to the sensory component of the nerve as well as the motor component in any surgical outcome analysis.

This chapter suggests a new facial nerve grading system that corrects these deficiencies. Table 2 delineates the classification with regard to the motor component of the facial nerve. Grades I and II, IV, V, and VI equate to the HB grades, but synkinesis and hemifacial spasm are graded separately. Moffat grade III is subdivided into A and B to take into account eye discomfort and exposure keratitis, which can have such a profound effect on quality of life. The grading of nervus intermedius or the sensory branch of the facial nerve

---

TABLE 2. Moffat facial nerve grading system (motor component of the facial nerve)

Moffat grade I equates to HB grade I
Moffat grade II equates to HB grade II
Moffat grade III is subdivided as follows:
    Grade III A: competent eye closure, eye comfortable and in good condition with or without lubricants
    Grade III B: competent eye closure, but eye dry and uncomfortable with evidence of exposure keratitis requiring lubricants and possibly medial or lateral tarsorrhaphy or a gold weight in the upper eyelid
Moffat grade VI equates to HB grade IV
Moffat grade V equates to HB grade V
Moffat grade VI equates to HB grade VI

HB, House–Brackmann

TABLE 3. Moffat facial nerve grading system (sensory: nervus intermedius function is classified with a suffix)

Crocodile tears (C)
   C0, no crocodile tears
   C1, crocodile tears present
Metallic or aberrant taste (T)
   T0, no aberrant taste
   T1, metallic or aberrant taste present
Dry eye (E)
   E0, no dry eye
   E1, dry eye present
Hemifacial spasm (H)
   H0, no hemifacial spasm present
   H1, hemifacial spasm present
Synkinesis (S)
   S0, no synkinesis present
   S1, synkinesis present

(Table 3) documents the patient's status with regard to crocodile tearing, metallic or aberrant taste, and dry eye, presented as a suffix, along with the presence or absence of hemifacial spasm and synkinesis.

For example, a patient with a Moffat grade III B—C1 T0 E1 H0 S1 would have good eye closure but an uncomfortable eye with exposure keratitis, crocodile tears, no taste abnormality, a dry eye, no hemifacial spasm, but synkinesis present. A patient with a Moffat grade II C0 T0 E0 H1 S1 would have almost normal facial movement with minimal asymmetry, no crocodile tears, no taste abnormality, no dry eye, but hemifacial spasm and synkinesis present.

This classification allows a comprehensive, accurate, and reliable assessment of the patient's facial nerve status in all respects.

References

1. Botman JWM, Jongkees LBW (1955) The results of intratemporal treatment of facial palsy. Pract Oto-Rhino-Laryngol 17:80–100
2. Janssen FP (1963) Ouvre de Postoperative Facialis-Verlamming. Thesis, University of Amsterdam, Amsterdam
3. May M (1970) Facial paralysis, peripheral type: a proposed method of reporting (emphasis on diagnosis and prognosis, as well as electrical and chorda tympani nerve testing). Laryngoscope 80(3):331–390
4. Adour KK, Swanson PJ Jr (1971) Facial paralysis in 403 consecutive patients with Bell's palsy. Trans Am Acad Ophthalmol Otolaryngol 75(6):1284–1301
5. Peitersen E (1977) Spontaneous course of Bell's palsy. In: Fisch U (ed) Facial nerve surgery, Zurich, 1976. Aesculapius, Birmingham, AL, pp 337–343

6. Yanagihara N (1977) Grading of facial palsy. In: Fisch U (ed) Facial nerve surgery. Proceedings, third international symposium on facial nerve surgery, Zurich, 1976. Aesculapius, Birmingham, AL, pp 533–535

7. Stennert E (1977) Facial nerve paralysis scoring system. In: Fisch U (ed) Facial nerve surgery. Proceedings, third international symposium on facial nerve surgery, Zurich, 1976. Aesculapius, Birmingham, AL, pp 543–547

8. House JW (1983) Facial nerve grading systems. Laryngoscope 93:1056–1069

9. Brackmann DE, Barrs DM (1984) Assessing recovery of facial function following acoustic neuroma surgery. Otolaryngol Head Neck Surg 92(1):88–93

10. House JW, Brackmann DE (1985) Facial nerve grading system. Otolaryngol Head Neck Surg 93:146–147

11. Burres SA, Fisch U (1986) The comparison of facial grading systems. Arch Otolaryngol Head Neck Surg 112:755–758

12. Murty GE, Diver JP, Kelly PJ, et al (1994) The Nottingham system: objective assessment of facial nerve function in the clinic. Otolaryngol Head Neck Surg 110(2):156–161

13. Chee GH, Nedzelski JM (2000) Facial nerve grading systems. Facial Plast Surg 16: 315–324

14. Croxon G, May M, Mester SJ (1990) Grading facial nerve function: House–Brackmann versus Burres–Fisch methods. Am J Otol 11(4):240–246

15. Evans RA, Haries ML, Baguley DM, et al (1989) Reliability of the House and Brackmann grading system for facial palsy. J Laryngol Otol 103(11):1056

16. Ross BG, Fradet G, Nedzelski JM (1996) Development of a sensitive clinical facial grading system. Otolaryngol Head Neck Surg 114(3):380–386

17. Rickenmann J, Jaquenod C, Cerenko D, et al (1997) Comparative value of facial nerve grading systems. Otolaryngol Head Neck Surg 117(4):322–325

18. Carmines EG, Zeller RA (1979) Reliability and valid assessment. In: Sage University paper series on quantitative applications in social sciences. Sage, Beverly Hills, pp 7–17

19. Landis JR, Koch GG (1977) The measurement of observer agreement for categorical data. Biometrics 33:159–174

20. Ahrens A, Skarada D, Wallace M, et al (1999) Rapid simultaneous comparison system for subjective grading scales for facial paralysis. Am J Otol 20:667–671

21. Irving RM, Viani L, Hardy DG, et al (1995) Nervus intermedius function after vestibular schwannoma removal: clinical features and pathophysiological mechanisms. Laryngoscope 105:809–813

22. Irving RM, Beynon GJ, Viani L, et al (1995) The patient's perspective after vestibular schwannoma removal: quality of life and implications for management. Am J Otol 16(3):331–337

Which International System Must be Chosen to Assess the Facial Function Before and After Acoustic Neuroma Treatment?

R. Charachon[1], J.P. Lavieille[1], and J.P. Chirossel[2]

Summary. The House–Brackmann grading system is used almost everywhere to assess post-treatment facial nerve function. However, the borders between grades I and II and between grades II and III may vary depending on the interpretation of the system and on the observer. This difficulty may undermine the reliability of reports on series. In the video and computer era, it seems inevitable to make a choice and to recommend one of the existing automatic systems of facial movement evaluation.

Key words. Facial function, Acoustic neuroma, Treatment

Since 1985, the House–Brackmann system of grading facial nerve recovery [1] has been adopted almost everywhere to assess the facial motricity after a facial paralysis or a treatment dealing with the facial nerve. Many other systems have been devised but only have a restricted use.

In the ENT Department of Grenoble University, 454 acoustic neuromas were operated on by the senior operator:

- 22 by suboccipital approach
- 369 by translabyrinthine approach
- 55 by retrosigmoid approach
- 8 by middle fossa approach

The large tumors, more than 3 cm (grade IV), were operated on by suboccipital approach up to 1982 by a team in which the neurosurgeon (Pr. De Rougemont) performed the largest part of the procedure, except drilling the

---

[1] ENT department, University of Grenoble, Chu Grenoble, BP 217, 38043 Grenoble, Cedex 09, France
[2] Neurosurgery Department, University of Grenoble, France

TABLE 1. Facial motoricity 1 year after surgery

Approach	House–Brackmann (HB) grade					
	HB I	HB II	HB III	HB IV	HB V	HB VI
Suboccipital (22)[a]	4%	9%	35%	48%	—	4%
Stage IV: 22						
Translabyrinthine (346)[b]	78%	12%	4%	3%	1%	2%
Stage I: 8						
Stage II: 189						
Stage III: 82						
Stage IV: 67						
Retrosigmoid (55)	89%	3.6%	3.6%	3.6%	0	0
Stage II: 51						
Stage III: 4						
Middle fossa (8)[c]	50%	12%	25%	12%	—	—
Stage I						

[a] In suboccipital approaches we classified:
  HB III: 1 end-to-end anastomosis
          1 hypoglossofacial anastomosis
  HB IV: 1 end-to-end anastomosis
          3 hypoglosso-facial anastomosis
[b] In translabyrinthine approaches we classified:
  HB III: 3 end-to-end anatomosis
          5 hypoglossofacial anastomosis
  HB IV: 3 end-to-end anastomosis
          4 hypoglosso-facial anastomosis
  HB V: 1 end-to-end anastomosis
  HB VI: 1 end-to-end anastomosis
[c] In retrosigmoid approaches we classified:
  HB IV: 1 hypoglossofacial anastomosis

internal auditory canal and dissection of the facial nerve in and around the canal. Since 1982, the large tumors were operated on by translabyrinthine approach, the otologist removing usually half the tumor (anterior part), followed by the neurosurgeon (Pr. Chirossel) removing the rest of the tumor. A total eradication was performed in all cases. The other tumors, those less than 3 cm, were usually removed by the otology team.

The final results on facial motoricity were assessed 1 year after surgery in 431 patients according to the House–Brackmann (HB) grading system (Table 1). We think 1 year is a good time limit because we observed, 3 years after surgery or later, slight synkinesis in patients having had a grade I without any postoperative deficit. Before 1985, the facial motoricity was expressed as a percentage according to an analytical system and then translated to a HB grading.

We could therefore observe the difficulties of the HB grading (Table 2): too much or too little in grade II and III. For grade II, the difficulty is "may have

TABLE 2. House–Brackmann system of grading facial nerve motoricity

Grade I: Normal
  Normal facial function in all areas.
Grade II: Mild dysfunction
  Gross: Slight weakness noticeable on close inspection. May have slight synkinesis.
  At rest, normal symmetry and tone.
  Motion: Forehead, moderate-to-good function.
  Eye, complete closure with minimal effort.
  Mouth, slight asymmetry.
Grade III: Moderate dysfunction
  Gross: Obvious but not disfiguring difference between two sides. Noticeable but not
    severe synkinesis, contracture or hemifacial spasm, or both.
  At rest, normal symmetry and tone.
  Motion: forehead, slight-to-moderate movement.
  Eye, complete closure with effort.
  Mouth, slightly weak with maximum effort.
Grade IV: Moderately severe dysfunction
  Gross: Obvious weakness or disfiguring asymmetry, or both.
  At rest, normal symmetry and tone.
  Motion: forehead, none.
  Eye, incomplete closure.
  Mouth, asymmetric with maximum effort.
Grade V: Severe dysfunction
  Gross: Only barely perceptible motion.
  At rest, asymmetry.
  Motion: forehead, none.
  Eye, incomplete closure.
  Mouth, slight movement.
Grade VI: Total paralysis
  No movement.

From [1], with permission

slight synkinesis". Some people do not admit any synkinesis at all in grade II. Nevertheless we never observed a grade II case without slight synkinesis 1 year after surgery. Grade III may have "noticeable but not severe synkinesis, contracture or hemifacial spasm or both." That is to say, a patient with grade III motricity with severe synkinesis or contracture has to be placed in grade IV. Nevertheless, it may be difficult to accurately distinguish slight, noticeable, and severe synkinesis. This distinction is not purely academic because good results on the facial nerve are classified I–II, or, sometimes, I–II–III (which is too much). It is very important to apply the grading correctly and to be objective, which can be difficult if the operating surgeon assesses the facial motricity.

For these reasons, we were fascinated by the Facial analysis Computerized evaluation (FACE) system (BioScan) developed by Neely and Cheung. The

Voluntary Motion

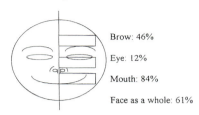

Brow: 46%

Eye: 12%

Mouth: 84%

Face as a whole: 61%

Associated Movements

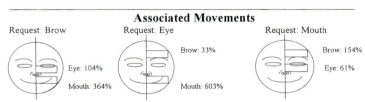

Request: Brow

Eye: 104%

Mouth: 364%

Request: Eye

Brow: 33%

Mouth: 603%

Request: Mouth

Brow: 154%

Eye: 61%

FIG. 1. Computerized analysis of a residual facial palsy after removing a left acoustic neuroma. Important synkinesis is seen at the mouth with voluntary motion of brow (364%) and eyelid (603%). There are also associated movements of the brow with contraction of the mouth (FACE System, 1997, BioScan)

Neely–Cheung FACE system measures differential light reflectance caused by facial surface deformation. At rest, the pixel gray scale values are established in the area of interest. In motion, they are substracted from each subsequent videoframe of the same area. It the area does not move, the substraction value is zero (black). If the area moves, the gray scale value is greater than zero: the more the area moves, the whiter the result. An intensity duration curve is thus produced and a program automatically calculates the contraction phase for each side, and for each specific facial region. The motion of the abnormal side is expressed as a percentage of the movement of the normal side. The score of the full half-face can also be assessed as a percentage. Synkinesis may be calculated as the excess motion compared to the normal side (Fig. 1).

In conclusion, in the computer era, automatic evaluation by a camera, a computer, and a program as developed by Neely et al. [2], Scriba et al. [3], or others [4] seems attractive. In the future, one system should be chosen to assess facial motricity.

References

1. House JW, Brackmann DE (1985) Facial nerve grading system. Otolaryngol Head Neck Surg 93:146–147
2. Neely JG, Joaquin AH, Kohn LA, et al. (1996) Quantitative assessment of the variation within grades of facial paralysis. Laryngoscope 106:438–442

3. Scriba H, Meier-Galati V, Fisch U (1997) An objective method of scaling facial function. In: 8th international symposium on the facial nerve, April 13–18, 1997, Matsuyama, Japan
4. Kawamoto M, Murata K, Isono M, et al. (1997) Computerized quantitative analysis of facial motion. In: Mc Cafferty G, Comand W, Carroll R (eds) XVI world congress of ORL head and neck surgery. Monduzzi, Rome, pp 103–111

Preservation of Facial Nerve Function After Acoustic Neuroma Surgery: Modification of the Facial Nerve Grading System

Chong Sun Kim[1], Sun O Chang[1], and Hee-Won Jung[2]

Summary. Facial nerve paralysis is a visible complication after acoustic neuroma surgery. In this study, the prognostic factors that can predict postoperative facial nerve function after acoustic neuroma surgery were investigated. The medical records of 68 patients with acoustic neuroma who underwent surgery with neurotological approaches from March 1987 to May 2001 at Seoul National University Hospital were reviewed retrospectively. The influence of surgical approach, preoperative facial nerve function, and tumor size on postoperative facial nerve function was determined by examining facial nerve function preoperatively, immediately postoperatively, and at the time of the last follow-up using the House–Brackmann grading system. Spearman correlation analysis was used for the statistical evaluation. Surgical approach for tumor removal and tumor extension had no influence on preserving the facial nerve. Preoperative and immediate postoperative facial nerve function and tumor size were important prognostic factors in long-term facial nerve function.

Key words. Facial nerve, Acoustic neuroma, Facial nerve grading system, Prognostic factor

Introduction

An acoustic neuroma is a benign tumor of the vestibular nerve. Facial nerve palsy is one of the most serious complications arising from acoustic neuroma surgery in the aspect of appearance. As the size of the tumor grows, a dys-

[1] Departments of Otolaryngology, [2] Departments of Neurosurgery, College of Medicine, Seoul National University, 28 Yeongon-dong, Chongno-gu, Seoul 110-744, Korea

function of the cochlear nerve and facial nerve palsy may occur. The reported cases of anatomic preservation of the facial nerve in acoustic neuroma surgery have been more than 90% [1]. However, preserving the function of the facial nerve is different from anatomic preservation. This study investigated the prognostic factors influencing postoperative facial nerve function.

Materials and Methods

This retrospective study included 68 patients who underwent surgery for acoustic neuroma between 1987 and 2001. The average age at the time of surgery was 50.7 years, ranging from 29 to 72 years. The average follow-up period was 28 months, ranging from 12 months to 9 years and 10 months. For total removal of the tumor mass at the skull base, the surgery was done in cooperation with a neurosurgeon.

The size of the acoustic neuroma was measured by magnetic resonance imaging (MRI) using the Guidelines of the Committee on Acoustic Neuroma. The axial MRI image showing the largest tumor size was selected, and only the extracanalicular portion of the tumor was measured. The first linear measurement was the diameter of the tumor in the direction parallel to the petrous ridge, and the second measurement was the maximum diameter of the tumor in orientation perpendicular to the first diameter. The tumor size was calculated as the square root of the product of these two diameters, and the result was rounded to the nearest 0.5 cm.

The surgical approach methods were selected according to the tumor location, size, the need to preserve hearing, and tumor extension such as intracanalicular or cerebellopontine angle extension. Facial nerve function was determined by examining the facial expression preoperatively, immediately postoperatively (7th day), and at the time of the last follow-up (>12 months) using the House–Brackmann grading system (HB grade). The tumor size was classified into five different groups: intracanalicular tumor and tumor sizes <10 mm, 10–25 mm, 26–40 mm, and >41 mm.

Tumor removal was also classified into four different categories. Gross total removal means removal of all the visible tumor, near-total removal means >95% removal of the tumor, subtotal removal means tumor removal of 50%–94%, and partial removal means <50%.

Statistical significance was determined using Spearman correlation analysis. To determine whether to reject the null hypothesis, a significance level of 0.05 was assumed for all calculations.

TABLE 1. Facial nerve preservation results ($n = 68$)

Pre-op		Immediate postop		Last F/U
HB grade	n (%)	HB grade	n (%)	n (%)
I–II	62 (91.2)	I–II	40 (64.5)	55 (88.7)
		III–IV	20 (32.3)	7 (11.3)
		V–VI	2 (3.2)	
III–IV	5 (7.3)	I–II	1 (20.0)	
		III–IV	2 (40.0)	4 (80.0)
		V–VI	2 (40.0)	1 (20.0)
V–VI	1 (1.5)	I–II		
		III–IV		
		V–VI	1 (100)	1 (100)

HB grade, House–Brackmann grade; Pre-op, preoperative; Immediate postop, postoperative 1 week; Last F/U, last follow-up at least 12 months postoperative

Results

Gross total removal of the tumor was performed in 64.7% of patients, near-total removal in 20.6%, subtotal removal in 8.8%, and partial removal in 5.9%. The translabyrinthine approach was selected in 45 cases, a transotic approach in 5, a middle fossa approach in 9, and a combined approach in 9 cases.

There was no significant difference between the preservation of facial nerve function and the approach method ($P > 0.05$). In addition, no correlation was found between extent of the tumor and facial nerve function ($P > 0.05$).

A significant difference was found between the end result of facial nerve function and facial nerve function at 1 week postoperative (Table 1). Furthermore, there was a statistically significant correlation between the tumor size and the preservation of facial nerve function. The larger the size of the tumor, the poorer the facial nerve function before surgery ($P < 0.05$) and at the last follow-up period ($P < 0.05$).

Discussion

The preservation of hearing and the functions of the facial nerve have been the most important concerns in acoustic neuroma surgery. An attempt was made to determine the prognostic factors influencing the preservation of facial nerve function after surgery. In this study, tumor size and facial nerve status 1 week after surgery were the most important prognostic factors predicting whether facial nerve function would be preserved. The presumed

TABLE 2. Moffat's modified House–Brackmann grade system

Grade IIIA
Competent eye closure
Eye comfortable/good condition with or without
lubricants
Grade IIIB
Competent eye closure
Dry eye/uncomfortable/exposure
keratitis/lubricants/tarsorrhaphy
Grade IV
Gross: obvious weakness
At rest: normal symmetry and tone
Forehead: none
Eye: incomplete closure
Mouth: asymmetry with maximal effort

mechanism of facial nerve injury associated with tumor size is as follows. The larger the tumor, the longer the surgical time needed and the larger the quantity of distorted anatomy. Therefore, more nerve injury can result.

With the recent development of MRI, an early diagnosis can be made even though the tumor is <1.0 cm in size. To preserve the function of the facial nerve, a short surgical duration and intact facial nerve anatomy are required. With smaller tumors, less adhesion with the adjacent tissue and less anatomic distortion occurs. Therefore, excising the tumor is easier and more of the facial nerve can be preserved.

Authors have been used the HB grading system and Fisch's scale system. In the Fisch system, eye closing was weighed as 30% of the total scale, same as the smiling motion, and forehead motion was weighed as only 10% of the total scale. In our facial nerve function study after acoustic nerve tumor surgery, the authors agreed to modify the HB grading system in two points.

First issue: grade III of the HB grading system is too broad, ranging from eye closure with minimum discomfort to severe eye sequelae such as exposure keratitis requiring possible tarsorrhapy. It is our suggestion to split this grade into IIIA and IIIB, as suggested by Dr. Moffat (Table 2), or to regrade the mild form of eye closure into grade III and the severe form into grade IV.

Second issue: forehead motion is weighed as only 10% of the total scale in Fisch's scale system. However, forehead motion in the HB grading system is overestimated, such as grade IV when there is no forehead motion. The authors' suggestion is to underestimate forehead function as grade III when forehead motion is absent. It could also be adopted in cases of facial nerve reanimation surgery, such as greater auricular nerve grafts or hypoglossal facial jump grafts, in which only grade IV with grade III facial nerve function is needed in all scales.

Reference

1. Hardy DG, Macfarlane R, Baguley D, et al. (1989) Surgery for acoustic neurinoma. An analysis of 100 translabyrinthine operations. J Neurosurg 71(6):799–804

Assessment of Facial Nerve Function Following Acoustic Neuroma Surgery: Facial Nerve Grading Systems

Naoaki Yanagihara and Naohito Hato

Summary. A number of grading systems for assessment of facial nerve function using gross or regional scales have been proposed internationally. At the Consensus Meeting of Acoustic Neuroma, the discussants agreed that the House-Brackmann scale was used most widely throughout the world, the Yanagihara system was always used in Japan and in some other countries, and other systems were used only by small groups. In view of the current situation, this chapter reviews the House-Brackmann scale and the Yanagihara system and describes the advantages and disadvantages of each system. The House-Brackmann grading scale is a representative gross scale that is useful for clinical purposes in general. However, all of the discussants agreed that the House-Brackmann scale needed to be modified to make it more relevant and reliable for assessing facial nerve function after acoustic neuroma surgery. The modification and its rationale are described. The Yanagihara system developed in Japan is a representative regional scale. The chart for obtaining the paralysis score is presented. The score provides accurate information on the grade of facial dysfunction to assess the course of recovery and to predict the outcome of the palsy. Conversion between the House-Brackmann scale and the Yanagihara paralysis score is described.

Key words. Grading system, Grading scale, Facial palsy, Facial nerve paralysis, Acoustic tumor surgery

Department of Otolaryngology, Ehime University School of Medicine, Shitsukawa, Shigenobu-cho, Onsen-gun, Ehime 791-0295, Japan

Introduction

International discussions on facial nerve grading scales and systems were first held at the Third International Symposium on Facial Nerve Surgery in Zurich in 1976 [1]. Since then, a number of grading systems have been proposed, and the issue of which is the most appropriate for evaluating facial nerve function was again discussed by the panels of the 1984, 1992, and 1997 International Symposia on the Facial Nerve. So far, none of these systems has been accepted for universal use.

The panel of the 1997 meeting held in Matsuyama City, Japan, recognized that the House-Brackmann scale was used most widely throughout the world, and that the Yanagihara system was always used in Japan and in some other countries. At the most recent Consensus Meeting of Acoustic Neuroma in 2001, the prevalence of the House-Brackmann scale and the Yanagihara system was again recognized. However, all of the discussants agreed that modification of the House-Brackmann scale was necessary, because the scale was inexact for assessing facial nerve function after acoustic neuroma surgery. Although the Japanese discussants were aware of the clinical value of the Yanagihara grading system, particularly its usefulness in the follow-up and prognosis of facial palsy, many of the non-Japanese invitees were unfamiliar with this system.

In view of this situation, this paper reviews the House-Brackmann scale and the Yanagihara system and describes how to use these systems to assess facial nerve function following acoustic neuroma surgery.

The House-Brackmann System

Facial grading scales or systems are divided into two major categories, the gross scale and the regional scale. Facial function has classically been divided into three grades: normal, partial palsy, and complete palsy. The gross scale is a continuation of the classical system. For example, in 1955, Botman and Jongkees used a five-point gross scale to describe the results of treatment of 70 patients with facial palsy (Table 1) [2]. Gross scales, as represented by that used by Botman and Jongkees, are designed to consider overall facial function and to describe the final outcome of the palsy. The observer is required to give one grade that presumably evaluates the degree of paralysis and secondary defects. The grades are arbitrary numbers in sequential order that proceed from the smallest deficit to the most severe deficit. Grading is a simple procedure that involves making a forced choice; however, facial palsy is a very complex phenomenon. Therefore, it is certain that there are patients for whom examiners reluctantly or with difficulty assign a single, definite grade. In such clinical situations, bias due to the nature of this choice may

TABLE 1. Botman-Jongkees classification

Class	Signification
O	Normal facial activity
I	Light paresis: normal at rest, talking normal, the eyes can be closed, some asymmetry in laughing and whistling
II	Moderate paresis: normal at rest, asymmetry in talking and laughing; the eyes cannot be closed
III	Severe paralysis: asymmetry at rest, dysfunction in movements
IV	Total paralysis: no tone, total loss of function. Contracture of the muscles may result in apparent improvement, and degeneration atrophy may cause a more serious aspect

result in disagreement as to the appropriate grade and may result in different choices among different examiners. Despite such uncertainties or inaccuracies, we must admit that the gross system is clinically useful, because grading can be done quickly without complex procedures and because the gross system provides common ground for assessing facial function and comparing the results of therapy.

Several other gross grading scales have been proposed. With the exception of the House-Brackmann scale, these have been used only by small groups. House studied the interobserver reliability of internationally proposed scales using videotaped recordings of patients' faces. Based on his findings, he designed a gross scale with six grades [3]. Each grade was well documented to help minimize interobserver disagreement and to ensure good reproducibility of results. Soon after the scale (Table 2) was introduced in 1983, the American Academy of Otolaryngology–Head and Neck Surgery accepted the scale as the reporting standard for facial palsy.

At the most recent consensus meeting, all of the invited discussants agreed that the House-Brackmann scale needed to be modified to make it more relevant and reliable for assessing facial nerve function after acoustic neuroma surgery. The proposed modifications were as follows: first, House-Brackmann grade III should be subdivided into subgrades A and B, where III-A indicates slight synkinesis and contracture, and III-B indicates moderate synkinesis and contracture; second, the at-rest component of grade IV should be changed to indicate asymmetry and weakness. Grade IV includes severe synkinesis and contracture.

The Yanagihara System

Regional scales for facial nerve function require the observer to independently score each different area of facial function and total all of the scores. The scores range either from 1 to 5 or from 1 to 3, or are based on percent-

TABLE 2. House-Brackmann facial nerve grading system

Grade	Description	Characteristics	
I	Normal	Normal facial function in all areas	
II	Mild dysfunction	Gross:	slight weakness noticeable only on close inspection; may have very slight synkinesis
		At rest:	normal symmetry and tone
		Motion:	Forehead: moderate to good function
		Eye:	complete closure with minimum effort
		Mouth:	slight asymmetry
III	Moderate dysfunction	Gross:	obvious but not disfiguring difference between two sides; noticeable but not severe synkinesis, contracture, and/or hemifacial spasm
		At rest:	normal symmetry and tone
		Motion:	Forehead: slight to moderate movement
		Eye:	complete closure with effort
		Mouth:	slight weakness with maximum effort
IV	Moderately severe dysfunction	Gross:	obvious weakness and/or disfiguring asymmetry
		At rest:	normal symmetry and tone
		Motion:	Forehead: none
		Eye:	incomplete closure
		Mouth:	asymmetric with maximum effort
V	Severe dysfunction	Gross:	only barely perceptible motion
		At rest:	asymmetry
		Motion:	Forehead: closure
		Eye:	incomplete closure
		Mouth:	slight movement
VI	Total paralysis	No movement	

ages of normal function. The scores are weighted when the examiner considers certain areas of the face to be more important for rating purposes. In contrast to the gross scale, the regional system requires both closer observation of the movement of each facial area and calculations to obtain a final score. However, once the examiner becomes familiar with the procedure, only a minute or two is required to obtain a final score.

Yanagihara, one of the authors, carried out a comparative study of gross and regional scales using videotaped recordings of patients' facial motions. From his results, he concluded that qualitative or descriptive scales were imprecise. He subsequently attempted to develop a more quantitative measuring tool [4–6].

As shown in Fig. 1, 10 discrete facial expressive states from 8 patients with facial palsies of various degrees and etiologies were videotaped under constant conditions to evaluate facial nerve function. Twelve facial nerve

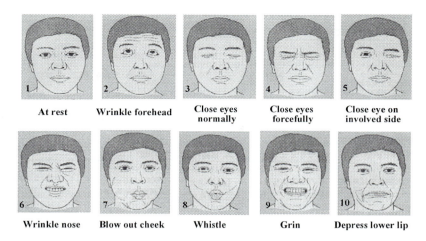

| At rest | Wrinkle forehead | Close eyes normally | Close eyes forcefully | Close eye on involved side |

| Wrinkle nose | Blow out cheek | Whistle | Grin | Depress lower lip |

FIG. 1. Ten discrete facial expressive states evaluated in the Yanagihara system

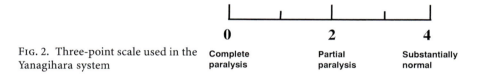

FIG. 2. Three-point scale used in the Yanagihara system

0 — Complete paralysis   2 — Partial paralysis   4 — Substantially normal

specialists graded each facial palsy using two scales; one was a five-point scale and the other was a three-point scale. On the five-point scale, 4 indicated normal expressive movements, and 3, 2, 1, and 0 indicated slight, moderate, severe, and total palsy, respectively (Fig. 2). On the three-point scale, 0 indicated total palsy, 2 indicated partial palsy, and 4 indicated normal function. The points given to each expressive state were added, and the total was called the paralysis score, which ranged from 40 (normal) to 0 (complete paralysis). The paralysis score was also expressed as a percentage (total points/40 × 100). No significant differences were seen between the paralysis scores obtained using the five-point scale and the three-point scale for each patient. However, the interjudge agreement for each facial expressive state was highest when the three-point scale was used. Therefore, a chart of the three-point scale of 10 facial expressive functions was designed because of its accuracy and clinical convenience (Fig. 3) [7].

The 40-point grading system has the following practical advantages: disturbances can easily be estimated from each expressive state without any confusion; all muscular functions required for emotional facial expression are included; the functional importance of the circumocular and circumoral muscles is adequately emphasized; facial expressive functions recovering

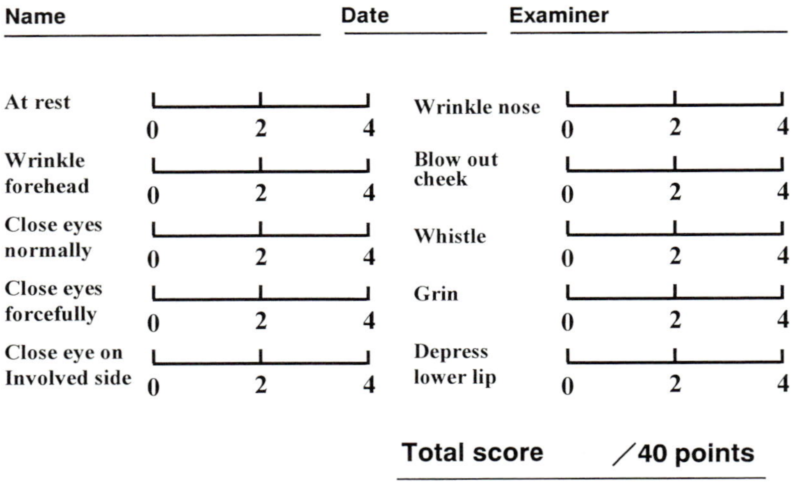

| Name | | Date | Examiner |

	0 2 4		
At rest	0 2 4	Wrinkle nose	0 2 4
Wrinkle forehead	0 2 4	Blow out cheek	0 2 4
Close eyes normally	0 2 4	Whistle	0 2 4
Close eyes forcefully	0 2 4	Grin	0 2 4
Close eye on Involved side	0 2 4	Depress lower lip	0 2 4

Total score   ╱40 points

FIG. 3. Chart of the three-point scales of 10 facial expressive functions used for calculating facial paralysis score

quickly and those recovering slowly from palsy are equally included with balance; and the clinical importance of loss of facial tone is brought to light. Continued studies on the reliability and clinical usefulness of this system were carried out between 1975 and 1980 by the Japanese Facial Nerve Study Group. The group subsequently accepted the Yanagihara 40-point scale as the Japanese standard for reporting the grade of facial palsy. So far, no opposition to this system has been voiced, nor have any modifications been advanced. A strong correlation between the Yanagihara score and integrated electromyographic recording has also been demonstrated [8]. A recent objective assessment of facial palsy using computerized image analysis of facial expressive movements and Moire topography also revealed that the paralysis score closely correlates with the objective score [9,10].

In this system, no special attention is paid to sequelae, such as synkinesis and contractures. We believe that each of the 10 facial expressive functions is disturbed to some extent by faulty regeneration of the facial nerve. The resultant dysfunction of the facial muscles is included in each rating score and is ultimately reflected in the paralysis score.

A conversion scale between the Yanagihara score and the House-Brackmann grade (H-B grade) was proposed by Satoh et al. (Table 3) [11]. A Yanagihara score of 40 approximates H-B grade I, 38–32 approximates grade II, 30–24 approximates grade III, 22–16 approximates grade IV, 14–8 approximates grade V, and 6–0 approximates grade VI. This conversion scale was approved by the Japanese Facial Nerve Study Group in 1995. Figure 4 shows

TABLE 3. Conversion between Yanagihara system and House-Brackmann system

Yanagihara system (points)	House-Brackmann system (grades)
40	I
32–38	II
24–30	III
16–22	IV
8–14	V
0–6	VI

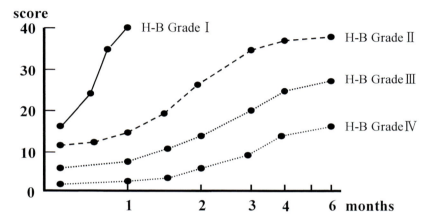

FIG. 4. Typical curves showing recovery of facial function obtained by the Yanagihara system

four typical examples of recovery curves for facial palsies obtained by the Yanagihara system. The outcomes of the facial palsies corresponded to H-B grades I, II, III, and IV. As shown here, examiners will be able to predict the course of recovery and will be able to determine the final outcome of the facial palsy when they become fully familiar with the Yanagihara system.

Comment

The House-Brackmann grading scale is a representative gross scale. It is very useful for clinical purposes, but slight modification of the scale is necessary to more accurately assess facial function after acoustic neuroma surgery. The Yanagihara system developed in Japan is a representative regional scale. It is easy to use and provides accurate information on the grade of dysfunction of the facial nerve and prediction of the outcome of the palsy.

References

1. Adour K (1977) Classification and standardized documentation of surgical results. In: Fisch U (ed) Facial nerve surgery. Proceedings: Third International Symposium on Facial Nerve Surgery, Zurich, 1976. Kugler Medical Publications, Amstelveen, Netherlands; and Aesculapius Publishing Co., Birmingham, AL, pp 527–554
2. Botman JWM, Jongkees LBW (1955) The results of intratemporal treatment of facial palsy. Pract Otorhinolaryngol 17:80–100
3. House JW (1983) Facial nerve grading systems. Laryngoscope 93:1056–1069
4. Yanagihara N, Kishimoto M (1972) Electrodiagnosis in facial palsy. Arch Otolaryngol 95:376–382
5. Yanagihara N, Nishimura H, Hazama K, et al. (1977) On standard documentation on facial palsy. Jpn J Otol Tokyo 80:21–27
6. Yanagihara N (1977) Grading of facial palsy. In: Fisch U (ed) Facial nerve surgery. Proceedings: Third International Symposium on Facial Nerve Surgery, Zurich, 1976. Kugler Medical Publications, Amstelveen, Netherlands; and Aesculapius Publishing Co., Birmingham, AL, pp 533–535
7. Yanagihara N (1985) Grading system for evaluation of facial palsy. In: Portman M (ed) Facial nerve. Proceedings: Fifth International Symposium on Facial Nerve, Bordeaux, 1984. Masson Publishing, New York, Paris, pp 41–42
8. Yagi S, Ishikawa Y (1980) Peripheral facial paralysis analyzed by integration of conventional EMG. Practica Otol, Kyoto 73:1355–1361
9. Kawamoto M, Isono M, Tanaka H, et al. (1995) Computerized quantitative analysis of facial motions: comparison with the Yanagihara's system. Facial N Res Jpn 15:81–84
10. Yuen K, Maeta M, Inokuchi I, et al. (1995) Evaluation of facial palsy by using the Moire topography index. Facial N Res Jpn 15:91–94
11. Sato Y, Kanzaki J, Yoshihara S (2000) A comparison and conversion table of the House-Brackmann facial nerve grading scale and the Yanagihara grading system. Auris Nasus Larynx 27:207–211

Part 3
Pre- and Postoperative Hearing

Patient Selection and Method of Evaluation for Hearing Preservation in Acoustic Neuroma Surgery

Takanori Fukushima

Summary. The goals of acoustic neuroma surgery are safe and accurate total tumor resection, normal facial nerve preservation, and hearing preservation. With the advances in extremely careful and meticulous microtechniques, hearing preservation has become possible in a high percentage of cases. This article deals with the criteria for patient selection in order to preserve good hearing function and discusses the key factors for hearing preservation and preoperative–postoperative evaluation of hearing function. Our criterion for selection of candidates for hearing preservation has been pure tone audiogram better than 50 dB loss and speech discrimination score better than 50 percent. This 50/50 criterion is still the standard; however, some patients with scores worse than 50/50 could be candidates for hearing preservation. Increasing clinical experience has indicated that the current American Academy of Otolaryngology–Head and Neck Surgery (AAO-HNS) hearing classification should be modified to divide C and D classes more precisely into several subtypes for better assessment of patient selection for hearing preservation.

Key words. Acoustic neuroma, Facial nerve, Hearing preservation, Vestibular nerve, Cochlear nerve

Duke University Medical Center, Director of Skullbase Surgery, Carolina Neuroscience Institute, Raleigh, North Carolina, 4030 Wake Forest Road, Suite 115 Raleigh, NC 27609, USA

Introduction

Surgery for acoustic neuromas is one of the most difficult in neurosurgery and in neuro-otology. In order to accomplish microsurgical total tumor resection for one-time cure in patients without any complications and to avoid palliative radiation therapy, the surgeon must have full understanding of temporal bone and cerebellopontine angle microanatomy and the most precise and sophisticated microtechnical skills, as well as abundant clinical experience. In recent years, operative results by expert teams have been markedly improved, with an incidence of facial nerve weakness of only a few percent, and currently world attention is focused upon the operative techniques of good hearing preservation in acoustic neuroma surgery. This chapter presents my experience with hearing preservation during the past two years, discussing the criteria for patient selection and the method of evaluation of operative results.

Clinical Materials and Patient Selection

From November 1998 until January 2001, I performed 63 consecutive unilateral acoustic neuroma surgeries at the Duke University Raleigh Hospital. Hearing preservation was attempted in 30 of these 63 patients. My previous experience with acoustic hearing preservation at Pittsburgh was published in *Laryngoscope* in 1997 [1], which defined candidates for hearing preservation surgery. The data showed that those patients who retained a pure tone audiogram (PTA) of less than 50 dB (1, 2, or 3 kHz) and a speech discrimination score (SDS) of greater than 50% in the preoperative condition had a good postoperative outcome for hearing preservation. This selection criterion can be applied for tumors smaller than 2.5 cm in diameter. If the acoustic neuroma becomes larger than 2.5 cm, the patient's preoperative hearing function needs to be better than 80% SDS in order to preserve usable hearing after surgery. The same criteria were used for the present series, but I added additional selection factors of identifiable wave-V in the preoperative auditory brainstem response (ABR) examination and the ability to carry on a telephone conversation using the affected ear.

Operative Technique

Acoustic neuromas confined to the internal auditory canal (IAC) or intrameatal mass plus small extrameatal extensions of less than 3 mm were resected by the middle fossa (MF) approach. The retrosigmoid approach (RS) was used for tumors exceeding 13 mm in the long axis. In all hearing preservation surgery, the tumor was removed with maximum careful, meticulous, and bloodless sharp microsurgical technique under continuous facial nerve and ABR monitoring. The intratumoral coring and debulking procedure is the important initial step, followed by medial to lateral tumor capsule elevation. Various sharp microdissectors, the 1-mm ring curette, the 1-mm cup curette, and the Storz Hitzelberger-McElveen knife are the key instruments for hearing preservation.

Results

The present series consisted of 16 men and 14 women ranging in age from 27 to 68 years (mean age, 49). The goals of each operation were total tumor removal, normal facial nerve function, and preservation of useful hearing. Total tumor resection was achieved in 27 patients (90%). I had to leave a small trace of thin capsule, like a little fingernail, in 3 patients who had larger tumors with capsules adherent to the cochlear nerve (near total resection, 10%). The cochlear nerve was anatomically well preserved in 28 cases (93.3%); however, ABR and good anatomical continuity were lost in 2 cases. Hearing function was evaluated by the classification of the American Academy of Otolaryngology–Head and Neck Surgery (AAO-HNS) Committee on Hearing and Equilibrium Guidelines [2]. The hearing level was reported as categories A, B, C, and D. Seventeen patients had class A hearing before surgery, and 6 patients retained class A level after surgery. Eight patients had class B hearing, and 3 patients went down to class D. Thirteen patients had class B hearing preoperatively; 1 patient improved to class A, 6 patients retained level B, 1 patient went down to class C, and 5 patients went down to class D. Overall, good hearing in classes A and B was preserved in 21 of 30 patients (70%). Among patients with still usable hearing in class C and some in class D, the hearing preservation rate went up to 80%. Hearing was preserved in 17 of 22 patients (77.3%) with tumors smaller than 20 mm and in 4 of 8 patients (50%) with tumors larger than 20 mm in diameter. Although the difference was not statistically significant, the hearing preservation rate appeared to be better in patients with tumors less than 20 mm in diameter.

Intraoperative ABR was performed in all cases, and we found that the preservation and maintenance of wave-V was significantly correlated with postoperative hearing preservation. In my experience, adhesion between the tumor capsule and the cochlear nerve is the most important factor for the preservation of hearing. In the present series, I noted 11 patients with severe adhesion and 19 without much fibrous adhesion. Hearing was preserved in only 2 of 11 patients with significant adhesion and in all 19 patients cases without much adhesion. There was no mortality or permanent complications in this series. One patient had postoperative CSF leak, which was resolved with conservative management. One patient required surgical debridement for wound infection.

Discussion

Controversy continues regarding patient selection for hearing preservation surgery and the criteria for defining success. It is generally accepted that hearing improvement in acoustic neuroma surgery is rare, but in the present series 4 patients gained improved hearing following the surgery. In my previous experience, I selected patients for hearing preservation with preoperative PTA less than 50 dB and SDS above 50%; however, increasing experience demonstrated that some patients with 60 dB loss and with good speech discrimination scores are still good candidates for hearing preservation. I have seen a few cases of hearing preservation even with preoperative speech discrimination scores of 30% to 40%.

The major problem of the AAO-HNS classification is that classes C and D are too broad. These categories should be classified into several subtypes of patients. For example, classes C and D should be divided into categories of patients with still usable hearing, serviceable hearing, any measurable hearing, and no hearing (deaf). In regard to the selection criteria based on tumor size, it is generally accepted that hearing preservation in patients with large tumors is very difficult and unlikely; however, during the past two decades I have preserved good hearing in 8 patients with tumors more than 3 cm in diameter and in many patients with tumors around 2 cm in diameter. As the present data indicate, the most important factor for hearing preservation is not tumor size but the surgeon's intraoperative finding of adhesion, because such fibrous adhesion hampers separation of the thin cochlear nerve from the tumor capsule. As to the selection of surgical approaches, my data show no statistically significant difference between the middle fossa approach and the retrosigmoid approach. The middle fossa approach has the significant disadvantages of longer operative time, more difficult exposure, longer hospital stay, and higher incidence of temporal lobe brain edema and temporary facial weakness. Even in cases of intrameatal tumor, I recommend increasingly that the operation should be performed through a simple retrosigmoid transmeatal approach.

Conclusion

The present study demonstrates that good hearing function can be preserved in more than 70% of cases with current meticulous microsurgical technique. Even with tumors over 2 cm in diameter, good hearing function can be achieved in 50% of cases. The present data showed that hearing was preserved in only 18% of cases with severe adhesion between the cochlear nerve and the tumor capsule, but in 100% of cases without severe adhesion. With further advances in neuroimaging technologies, preoperative evaluation of fibrous adhesion between the tumor capsule and the remaining nerve may become possible and, hopefully, will result in good selection of patients for hearing preservation surgery. Increasing clinical experience demonstrates that even some patients in classes C and D can be candidates for hearing preservation and that these patients can still have useful postoperative hearing levels. The current AAO-HNS hearing classification should be modified to divide classes C and D into several subtypes for better assessment of patient selection criteria and postoperative outcome.

References

1. Arriaga MA, Chen DA, Fukushima T (1997) Individualizing hearing preservation in acoustic neuroma surgery. Laryngoscope 107:1043–1047
2. Committee on Hearing and Equilibrium (1995) Committee on Hearing and Equilibrium guidelines for the evaluation of hearing preservation in acoustic neuroma (vestibular schwannoma). Otolaryngol Head Neck Surg 113:179–180

Some Proposals on Reporting Systems in Acoustic Neuroma

Jin Kanzaki, Takanobu Kunihiro, and Yasuhiro Inoue

Summary. Some proposals on reporting systems regarding tumor size, pre- and postoperative hearing results, tinnitus, and equilibrium disorder have been suggested.

1. Tumor size: Six grades including intracanalicular and five 10-mm sections together with tumor characteristics (solid or cystic) and the absence or the presence of fundus invasion have been proposed.
2. Hearing: We recommended that pure tone hearing level and the speech discrimination score should be reported separately because considerable discrepancies are often seen between them.
3. Tinnitus: Loudness of pre- and postoperative tinnitus and annoyance caused by tinnitus and evaluation of each change should be assessed independently and separately.
4. Vertigo and disequilibrium: Grading of pre- and postoperative vertigo and disequilibrium, and evaluation of change in vertigo and disequilibrium were proposed.

Key words. Acoustic neuroma, Reporting system, Preoperative hearing, Postoperative hearing, Tinnitus, Vertigo

Introduction

The importance of the standardization of reporting results has been emphasized since the first Acoustic Neuroma Conference in Copenhagen held in 1991, and even at the recent conference in Rome in June 1999. However, as

Department of Otolaryngology, School of Medicine, Keio University, 35 Shinanomachi, Shinjuku-ku, Tokyo 160-8582, Japan

always, the main problem is that the time allotted to discuss these evaluation methods is too short. We hope, in this conference, that reporting systems on the results of acoustic neuroma will be discussed and gain consensus at a future conference.

We would like to suggest our ideas on some of the reporting systems for tumor size, evaluation of pre- and postoperative hearing results, pre- and postoperative tinnitus, and equilibrium disorders.

Measurement of Tumor Size

In surgery for acoustic neuromas, tumor size greatly influences the postoperative condition (e.g., hearing, facial nerve function). Therefore, a common reporting system for tumor size should be established. (This concept is not intended to prohibit individual institutes from using their own method for research work.)

The most commonly used methods for reporting tumor size include a, $a \times b$, and $\sqrt{a \times b}$, where a and b are the length of the tumor along the axis parallel and perpendicular to the internal auditory canal, respectively. Although still controversial, the first method seems to be most clinically relevant.

When we want to measure the diameter along the internal auditory canal (IAC), it is clear to everyone where we should measure. The relation of the size of the tumor to the brainstem is well understood. On the other hand, $a \times b$ may correspond to a tumor volume. When using the greatest diameter, we do not know in which direction a tumor should be measured. Without being able to do this, we cannot get a picture of the relation of the tumor to the brainstem. Using the first method, tumor size is usually classified into the following five categories:

Intracanalicular
Small   Extending 15 mm or less into the posterior fossa
Medium   Extending 16–25 mm into the posterior fossa
Large   Extending 26–40 mm into the posterior fossa
Giant   Extending 41 mm or more into the posterior fossa

However, this classification does not work properly, because (1) a small tumor is defined as 15 mm or less in size (this is too large), and (2) hearing preservation surgery is generally performed for tumors 20 mm (not 15–25 mm) or less in size. We propose the following classification, which defines tumor size every 10 mm:

I (intracanalicular)
II (small)   Extending 10 mm or less into the posterior fossa
III (medium)   Extending 11–20 mm into the posterior fossa

IV (moderately large)   Extending 21–30 mm into the posterior fossa
V (large)   Extending 31–40 mm into the posterior fossa
VI (giant)   Extending 41 mm or more into the posterior fossa

It is preferable to describe tumor size together with its characteristics (solid or cystic) and the presence or absence of fundus invasion. A small tumor not invading the fundus, for example, can be described as II-M (M means medial). If the tumor is solid, it can be described as II-MS (S, solid). In the same way, a cystic medium-sized tumor not invading the fundus can be described as III-MC (C, cystic).

Evaluation of Pre- and Postoperative Hearing Results

The indication of hearing preservation surgery should be mainly based on tumor size, preoperative hearing level, and speech discrimination score. In addition, hearing level in the contralateral ear is also taken into consideration.

Hearing preservation surgery is not usually attempted for patients with a large tumor; the majority of otoneurosurgeons consider that hearing preservation surgery should be attempted only for patients with tumors less than 20 mm in diameter. In addition, patients with poor preoperative hearing should also be excluded from candidates for hearing preservation surgery, because hearing that has deteriorated before the operation rarely improves after tumor removal.

The classification proposed by AAO-HNS is an excellent grading system of hearing. However, we would like to amend it for the following reasons.

1. In this system, hearing level is calculated at frequencies of 0.5, 1, 2, and 3 kHz. However, hearing at 3 kHz is not measured routinely in Japan. Therefore, it would be more convenient if the hearing level at 4 kHz were used instead of that at 3 kHz.

2. Vestibular schwannoma (VS) has been diagnosed in patients having normal hearing in recent years. In these cases, it is important to know in advance whether hearing can be preserved. We consider that "normal" hearing should fulfill both the following two criteria: (1) pure tone average (PTA) hearing level ≤ 20 dB, and (2) speech discrimination score (SDS) $\geq 80\%$. We also recommend that pure tone hearing level and SDS should be reported separately, because considerable discrepancies are often seen between them. We think that Sanna's grade V and VI could be excluded because patients with these preoperative grades are not indicated for hearing preservation surgery.

PTA
- I: 0–20 dB
- II: 21–40 dB
- III: 41–60 dB
- IV: 61 dB–

SDS
- A: 100%–80%
- B: 79%–60%
- C: 59%–40%
- D: 39%–

According to this new reporting system, hearing would be reported as I-A, II-C, IV-D, as appropriate.

3. In the AAO-HNS system, there is no definition of the time to evaluate post-operative hearing. The hearing level usually changes during several months after tumor removal because of middle ear effusion, change in cochlear microcirculation, and damage to the cochlear nerve itself. Therefore, we propose to determine the time to evaluate postoperative hearing. We think it appropriate to report hearing measured 6 months after surgery.

Evaluation of Pre- and Postoperative Tinnitus

Tinnitus is one of the most common symptoms of acoustic neuromas and affects the patient's quality of life considerably. Therefore, a concise, practical grading system for tinnitus is imperative. We propose the following scales to assess pre- and postoperative tinnitus.

Loudness of pre- and postoperative tinnitus:
- I.   No tinnitus
- II. The ear sometimes rings during silence
- III. The ear always rings during silence
- IV. Tinnitus is always present

Annoyance caused by pre- and postoperative tinnitus:
- I.   No tinnitus (no annoyance)
- II. Tinnitus is present, but does not cause a problem in daily activities
- III. No problem when concentrating on work
- IV. Cannot concentrate on work
- V.   Cannot get to sleep because of tinnitus
- VI. Chronic insomnia

The loudness of pre- and postoperative tinnitus should be assessed independently (e.g., grade II → grade III). The degree of annoyance should also be assessed independently (e.g., grade III → grade V). Based on these results, the influence of surgery on tinnitus is graded as follows:

Change in loudness:

Markedly improved	Improved by three grades
Moderately improved	Improved by two grades
Slightly improved	Improved by one grade
Unchanged	No change
Slightly aggravated	Worsened by one grade
Moderately aggravated	Worsened by two grades
Markedly aggravated	Worsened by three grades

Change in annoyance:

Markedly improved	Improved by three grades or more
Moderately improved	Improved by two grades
Slightly improved	Improved by one grade
Unchanged	No change
Slightly aggravated	Worsened by one grade
Moderately aggravated	Worsened by two grades
Markedly aggravated	Worsened by three grades or more

Assessment of Vertigo and Disequilibrium

Acoustic neuromas arise from the vestibular branches of the VIIIth cranial nerve. However, vertigo attacks and disequilibrium are seen in only 20% of patients preoperatively, presumably because of the slow progress of vestibular nerve dysfunction and associated compensation by the central nervous system.

In acoustic neuromas, two types of pathophysiology can explain the occurrence of vertigo and disequilibrium: (1) acute exacerbation of vestibular nerve function, and (2) compensation by the brainstem and cerebellum. The former is thought to occur as a result of compromised circulation to the nerve and inner ear.

Based on these considerations, we propose the following grading system for pre- and postoperative balance disorder:

<Grading of pre- and postoperative vertigo/disequilibrium>

Grade	Definition
I	No symptom
II	Mild dizziness (floating sensation) with/without transient vertigo
III	Moderate to severe dizziness (floating sensation) or severe, recurrent vertigo attacks
IV	Mild truncal ataxia
V	Moderate to severe truncal ataxia

<Change in vertigo/disequilibrium>

Markedly relieved	Improved by two or more grades
Moderately relieved	Improved by one grade
Unchanged	No change
Moderately aggravated	Worsened by one grade
Markedly aggravated	Worsened by two or more grades

Outcome Reporting in Hearing Preservation Surgery: The Place of the MRI Follow-Up

A. Mazzoni[1], V. Calabrese[1], and R. Barbò[2]

Summary. The problem of a potential residual or recurrent acoustic neuroma in the hearing preservation procedure was investigated in a series of 230 consecutive cases that were submitted to a longtime Gd-MRI protocol. The rate of follow-up was 96.9%. It is suggested that clinical reports on the outcome of hearing preservation procedures include a long-term protocol with Gd-MRI at postoperative intervals of 1, 3, 6, and 10 years.

Key words. Hearing preservation, Acoustic neuroma, MRI follow-up

Introduction

Magnetic resonance imaging with gadolinium-DTPA (Gd-MRI) is currently the most accurate method for detecting small intracanalicular neuromas of nerve VIII or residual or recurrent tumors after hearing preservation surgery. Functional procedures for acoustic neuroma removal entail a risk of recurrent pathology, either from remnants of tumor left in the lateral end of the internal auditory canal (residual tumor) or from the preserved nerves because of late degeneration (recurrent tumor).

This study of a series of 230 acoustic neuroma cases operated on with a hearing preservation procedure involved a long-term Gd-MRI control and suggests a method of follow-up. The MRI follow-up includes typical images for tumor, typical images for nontumor, histological validation of images, time between surgery and significant images, time-related changes in tumor and nontumor images, and time required to rule out residual tumor. A follow-up

[1] Department of Otorhinolaryngology, [2] Department of Neuroradiology, Ospedali Riuniti, Bergamo, Italy

protocol in an ordinary, noninvestigational setting for residual and recurrent tumor is proposed.

Materials and Methods

During the period from 1976 to 2000, 230 consecutive patients with acoustic neuroma underwent operation in our department. The surgical procedure for total tumor removal was performed by the same surgeon via a suboccipital transmeatal approach without or with direct exposure of the lateral end of the internal auditory canal, respectively, in 86 (1976–1992) and 144 (1992–2000) cases. Our protocol included Gd-MRI at 1, 3, 5, and 8 years after surgery or yearly MRI if the patient showed any change in postoperative hearing and in MRI-positive cases.

MRI investigations were carried out in our institution in the majority of cases (58%) using the same scanner (Sigma-GE, 1.5 Tesla Imager) and the same sequences (axial and coronal T1-weighted images, with a relaxation time of 500 ms, an echo time of 25 ms, and contiguous slice thickness of 3 mm), without and with intravenous administration of contrast material (gadolinium) at a standard dose of 0.1 mmol/kg. In the other 48% of the cases, the same team reviewed the images submitted from other neuroradiological centers. Postoperative MRI with gadolinium (i.e., baseline MRI) was performed in 223 cases (96.9%); in the remaining 7 cases this was not possible because of 2 deaths, 3 refusals, and 2 MRIs without gadolinium. MRI features were classified according to criteria reported in Table 1 (a and b).

Results

Analysis of postoperative MRI (at the last follow-up examination) revealed four distinct pictures (Table 2).

Based upon the two main phases of the evolution of our surgical technique (1976–1992, without fundus exposure; 1992–2000, with fundus exposure), results are reported in Tables 3 and 4.

Unspecific enhancement (E+) was apparent at the first or second MRI and faded away in half of the cases, that is, in one quarter within the third postoperative year and one quarter within 10 years; the remaining half had no changes. Possible or suspected tumor (E++) was apparent in 4 patients. It slowly disappeared within 5 to 10 years in 3 cases and remained stable in 1 case. The total recurrence/residual rate was to 2.2%, and all the five cases with recurrent/residual pathology were apparent in the group of 79 patients operated on without direct access to the fundus. The history of these five recurrences is shown in Table 5.

TABLE 1. Evaluation criteria in MRI Gd-DTPA follow-up

a) Enhancement
    Enhancement + (artefacts, nerve edema, scar tissue, tumor)
        Location (within the operative site)
            At the fundus of the internal auditory canal
            Along the course of the acousticofacial bundle
            Along the borders of the meatal bone resection
        Appearance
            Nodular
            Linear
        Size change with time

b) No enhancement
    Enhancement + not significant for tumor
        Round in shape, but decreasing with time
        Linear in shape
    Enhancement ++ for presumed tumor
        Ø > 3 mm, stable in time, round in shape, located in the internal auditory canal
    Enhancement +++ for certain tumor
        Ø > =3 mm
        Ø < 3 mm and size increase with time

TABLE 2. Gd-MRI results in suboccipital removal of acoustic neuroma (N = 223/230)

No enhancement	203
Enhancement + (unspecific enhancement)	14
Enhancement ++ (possible tumor)	1[a]
Enhancement +++ (tumor)	5[b]

[a] Possible tumor, stable for 10 years
[b] Proven at revision surgery

TABLE 3. Gd-MRI follow-up in retrosigmoid approach without fundus exposure (1976–1992) (N = 79; range, 8–17 years; average, 10 years)

No enhancement	64	(6 previous E+; 2 previous E++)
Enhancement + (unspecific enhancement)	9	(3 operated on to control histology of image)
Enhancement ++ (possible tumor)	1[a]	(2 regressed to no enhancement)
Enhancement +++ (tumor)	5	(all operated on and histologically confirmed)

[a] At postoperative year 10: stable image and good hearing

Table 4. Gd-MRI follow-up in retrosigmoid approach with fundus exposure (1992–2000) (N = 144; range, 1–9 years; average, 5 years)

No enhancement	139	(9 previous E+; 1 previous E++)
Enhancement + (unspecific enhancement)	5	
Enhancement ++ (Possible tumor)	0	(1 regressed to no enhancement)
Enhancement +++ (tumor)	0	

TABLE 5. "History" of recurrence cases. (N = 5/223)

Patient	Time postoperation (yr)	Ø (mm)	Site	Management
A.A.	6	2		
	7	3	Fundus	Surgery
C.L.	7	15	IAC + CPA	Surgery
F.A.	7	15	IAC + CPA	Surgery
M.M	5	9	IAC	Surgery
M.R.	5	3	Fundus	Surgery

IAC, internal auditory canal; CPA, cerebellopontine angle

Conclusions

The present study assessed the nature of Gd-MRI images of surgical speci-
mens. A linear, stable, or decreasing enhancement image indicated unspecific
scar tisssue; a nodular, stable, or increasing image was typical of tumor. The
time between surgery and the MRI finding of the smallest (2-mm) tumor was
6 years. Nontumor images disappeared in time in over half of the cases.

It is proposed that a postoperative follow-up protocol should include
Gd-MRI at intervals of 1, 3, 6, and 10 years. If a lesion typical of small tumors
(≤ 2 mm in diameter) is found, further management should include a yearly
MRI check in order to plan the most appropriate treatment. An outcome
study should group separately tumors assessed from the surgical specimen
and cases diagnosed only by Gd-MRI.

References

1. Mazzoni A, Calabrese V, Moschini L (1996) Residual and recurrent acoustic neuroma in
   hearing preservation procedures: neuroradiologic and surgical findings. Skull Base Surg
   6:105–112
2. Mazzoni A, Calabrese V, Danesi G (2000) A modified retrosigmoid approach for direct
   exposure of the fundus of the internal auditory canal for hearing preservation in
   acoustic neuroma surgery. Am J Otol 21:98–109
3. Sekiya T, Suzuky S, Iwabuchi T (1990) Changes in intracochlear and intracanalicular
   nerves after acoustic neurinoma excision confirmed by magnetic resonance imaging.
   Neurosurgery 27:587–591
4. Thedinger B, Whittaker C, Luetje C (1991) Recurrent acoustic tumor after a suboccipital removal. Neurosurgery 29:681–687
5. Thomassin JM, Pellet W, Epron JP, Braccini F, Roche PH (2001) Les récidives des neuri-
   nomes de l'acoustique après exérèse chirurgicale. Ann Otolaryngol Chir Cervicofac
   118(1):3–10

New Classification of Postoperative Hearing Results Following Acoustic Neuroma Surgery

Shingo Murakami, Nobuhiro Watanabe, and Sotaro Kamei

Summary. The classification system of the Committee on Hearing and Equilibrium of the American Academy of Otolaryngology–Head and Neck Surgery (AAO–HNS) is currently used to evaluate postoperative hearing results. This system is suitable for evaluating patients who have useful preoperative hearing of class A or B. However, the system is not suitable for evaluating patients who have poor hearing of class C or D. To evaluate both patients with good and those with poor preoperative hearing, we propose the following new evaluation system. Unchanged: postoperative hearing change is less than 15 dB-15%. Improved: postoperative hearing is improved more than 20 dB-20%. Worse: postoperative hearing is decreased more than 20 dB-20%.

Key words. Acoustic neuroma surgery, Middle cranial fossa approach, Hearing preservation, Evaluation of postoperative hearing

Introduction

The postoperative hearing result as well as facial nerve function is a important indicator for evaluating surgical intervention in acoustic neuroma. The classification system of the Committee on Hearing and Equilibrium of the American Academy of Otolaryngology–Head and Neck Surgery (AAO–HNS) [1] is currently used to evaluate postoperative hearing results. This system includes both pure tone hearing thresholds and speech discrimination score and classifies hearing into four grades: classes A, B, C, and D. This system is

Department of Otolaryngology, Nagoya City University, Medical School, 1 Kawasumi Mizuho-cho, Mizuho-ku, Nagoya 467-8601, Japan suitable for evaluating patients who have useful preoperative hearing of class A or B. However, the system is not suitable for evaluating patients who have poor hearing of classes C and D. We occasionally do hearing preservation surgery in selected patients with sudden onset of severe hearing loss, because their hearing sometimes improves after tumor resection. Therefore, another classification system for both patients with good and those with poor preoperative hearing is desired.

In the present study, we analyze pre- and postoperative hearing in 63 cases of acoustic neuroma operated via the middle cranial fossa approach, and we propose a new classification system.

Materials and Methods

Sixty-three patients underwent acoustic neuroma surgery via the middle cranial fossa approach at the hospitals of Ehime University and Nagoya City University. Thirty had intracanalicular tumors, 28 had small tumors, and 5 had medium-sized tumors. In the present study, we propose the following new evaluation system for postoperative hearing results. Unchanged: postoperative hearing change is less than 15 dB-15%. Improved: postoperative hearing is improved more than 20 dB-20%. Worse: postoperative hearing is decreased more than 20 dB-20% (Table 1).

Results and Comments

Pre- and postoperative hearing results were evaluated both by the AAO–HNS system and by our new classification system. Figure 1 shows the results of hearing preservation in patients whose preoperative hearing was in classes A and B. Twenty-nine patients were in class A and 22 were in class B preoperatively. Among 51 patients in class A or B, 34 remained in class A or B. However, 17 patients deteriorated to class C or D postoperatively. According to our evaluation system, improvement was seen in 1 patient, 33 were unchanged, and 17 were worse (Fig. 1). On the other hand, among 12 patients with class C or D preoperative hearing, 9 patients remained in class C or D, but 3 patients improved to class B postoperatively (Fig. 2). According to our system, improvement was seen in 2 patients, 7 patients were unchanged, and 3 patients were worse (Fig. 2).

TABLE 1. New classification of postoperative hearing results

Improved: Improved more than 20 dB-20%
Unchanged: Change is less than 15 dB-15%
Worse: Decreased more than 20 dB-20%

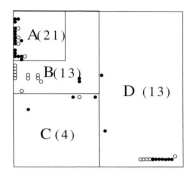

	No of Cases
Improved	1 (2%)
Unchanged	33 (65%)
Worse	17 (33%)

FIG. 1. Postoperative hearing results in patients with preoperative class A (*filled circles*) or class B (*open circles*) hearing ($n = 51$)

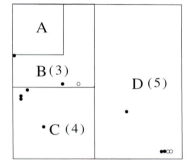

	No of Cases
Improved	2 (17%)
Unchanged	7 (58%)
Worse	3 (25%)

FIG. 2. Postoperative hearing results in patients with preoperative class C (*filled circles*) or class D (*open circles*) hearing ($n = 12$)

In acoustic neuroma surgery, hearing preservation is generally indicated in patients who have useful preoperative hearing of class A or B. Consequently, the success of surgery is evaluated only according to how many patients with useful hearing remain in class A or B postoperatively. However, an evaluation system is needed even for patients with poor preoperative hearing, because hearing improvement is occasionally seen after tumor resection [2]. Moreover, the AAO-HNS system is not suitable for evaluating the success of surgery. For example, if postoperative hearing is restored within the same class (A to A or B to B), can we recognize this operation as successful? Conversely, if postoperative hearing changes from class A to class B or from class B to class C, can we recognize this operation as not successful? That is, if preoperative hearing of 30 dB-70% (class A) deteriorates to 40 dB-60% (class B), can we recognize this operation as not successful? On the other hand, even if preoperative hearing of 0 dB-100% (class A) is restored within the same class A to 30 dB-70%, can we recognize this operation as successful? To resolve this dilemma, we have proposed new criteria of "unchanged, improved, and worse." In our system, a successful operation may belong to the "unchanged" group and an unsuccessful operation to the "worse" group. Although hearing improvement after acoustic neuroma surgery is quite rare, we may call this result "excellent." This system is available for patients with either good or poor preoperative hearing and correlates well with the AAO-HNS system.

References

1. Committee on Hearing and Equilibrium guidelines for the evaluation of hearing preservation in acoustic neuroma (vestibular schwannoma) (1995) Otolaryngol Head Neck Surg 113:179–180
2. Yanagihara N, Murakami S (1998) Preservation and improvement of hearing following surgical removal of small acoustic tumor. Neurologia 38:605–606

Sense and Nonsense of Hearing After Vestibular Schwannoma Surgery

BERNARD K.H. PAUW[1] and CEES J.J. AVEZAAT[2]

Summary. Hearing preservation (HP) remains a challenge in vestibular schwannoma treatment. The literature and the authors' experience are reviewed. Classification of hearing is essential. The American Academy of Otolaryngology–Head and Neck Surgery (AAO-HNS) classification is a major improvement. From 12 surgical series, only 16% of patients were actual candidates for HP. The average HP rate in patients with small tumors and class A or B hearing was 42% (808 attempted cases). When all tumor sizes and hearing levels were considered, the HP rate was 38% (2751 attempted cases). Delayed hearing loss was found in 19% after a mean follow-up period of 4.6 years. The AAO-HNS classification lacks a definition of time interval for postoperative audiometry. Moreover, the pure tone average (PTA) in the literature is not calculated in a uniform way. We conclude that the probability of lasting HP is not more than 0.35. Audiometry at 1 year post-treatment should be included in HP reports. A uniform way of calculating PTA is recommended.

Key words. Vestibular schwannoma, Acoustic neuroma, Hearing preservation, Hearing classification

Introduction

The number of patients suitable for conservation of hearing function varies between 1% and 10% of the total population with vestibular schwannoma, depending on the criteria used [1]. The usefulness of residual hearing re-

---

[1]ORL Department H 895, [2]Department of Neurosurgery, Erasmus MC, Postbox 2040, 3000 CA Rotterdam, The Netherlands

mains a much-debated issue. Critical reviews are reported by Gardner and Robertson [2], Shelton [3], Whittaker and Luetje [4], Glasscock et al. [5], and Sanna et al. [6]. With the advent of stereotactic irradiation, the question is raised as to whether hearing is really that important, given the treatment options: observation, irradiation, and operation. This report is a literature study on hearing preservation (HP) after vestibular schwannoma surgery, focusing on reporting hearing results.

Classification of Hearing

In many reports, the so-called 50/50 rule of Wade and House [7] is used for the definition of serviceable or useful hearing, meaning a pure tone average (PTA) ≤ 50 dB and speech discrimination score (SDS) ≥ 50%. Whittaker and Luetje [4] and Glasscock et al. [5] are of the opinion that for a successful HP, the operated side must maintain a hearing level that can be substantially improved with a conventional hearing aid, which implies a PTA of at least 70 dB and a SDS of more than 70%.

In 1995 the Committee on Hearing and Equilibrium of the American Academy of Otolaryngology–Head and Neck Surgery (AAO-HNS) [8] proposed an ABCD classification system for the assessment of hearing in the treatment of vestibular schwannomas. These standards should make it possible to compare published results and to evaluate the effectiveness of selection procedures, surgical techniques, and monitoring. Even with the use of a uniform grading system, one should be on the alert for pitfalls. Five ways of calculating the PTA can be found in the literature, which differ in both the number and the levels of thresholds taken into account.

Review of Literature on Vestibular Schwannoma Surgery

Gardner and Robertson [2] compiled the results of 11 surgical series, including 404 patients, limited to unilateral vestibular schwannomas, providing evidence of valid postoperative audiometry and defining success in terms of the least stringent criteria. They reported a success rate of 33%. Shelton [3] found measurable postoperative hearing in 12% to 65% of patients in 10 published series from the literature. In the studies reporting such data, hearing was preserved near the preoperative level in 21% to 35% of cases.

The results, in relation to tumor size, from 12 series [9–18] including 4287 patients were studied. Only 16% of patients were actual candidates for HP. The average HP rate was 42% (808 attempted cases). Shelton and House [19] reported hearing improvement in 8.5% of patients undergoing attempted HP. A postoperative decline in hearing over the years is a more frequent occurrence. Although Rosenberg et al. [20] found no significant hearing loss over a follow-up period of 1.3 to 11 years in 9 patients, several authors did report worsening of hearing after initial successful preservation. Approximately one-half of 25 patients of Shelton et al. [21], followed for 3 to 20 years, suffered a significant decrease of hearing in the operated ear, with a mean loss of 12 dB in PTA and of 25% in SDS. McKenna et al. [22] found a significant decline in hearing in 4 of 18 patients (22%) after 3 to 10 years. Umezu et al. [23] followed up 17 patients with retained hearing in the early postoperative period for more than 6 months and reported that hearing declined at a PTA of 25 dB or more in 3 patients. In our own series, 226 patients with 229 tumors underwent operation from 1982 to 1999. HP was attempted in patients with small tumors and useful hearing only, that is, class A and B. In 14 of 25 patients (56%), hearing was retained. The mean follow-up was more than 2 years. On average, the pure tone average declined from 28 to 37 dB and the mean speech discrimination score decreased from 95% to 86%.

Discussion

Twelve series from the literature, including 4287 patients, were analyzed for potential candidates for HP. Taking into account hearing level (class A or B) and tumor size (<15 mm extrameatal), only 16% of patients were actual candidates for HP. The average HP rate in patients with small tumors and class A or B hearing was 42% (808 attempted cases). The authors' HP rate was 56%. When all tumor sizes and hearing levels were considered, the HP rate was 38% (2751 attempted cases). The AAO-HNS hearing classification is a major improvement in the reporting of hearing results after vestibular schwannoma treatment. However, a definition of the time after the operation at which audiometry should be performed is lacking. Long-term hearing deterioration implies that HP results should include pure tone and speech audiometry data 1 year after the operation. Moreover, PTA in the literature is not always calculated in the same way. International consensus in this matter is needed.

Conclusion

The probability of lasting hearing preservation is not more than 0.35. Audiometry at 1 year post-treatment should be included in HP reports. A uniform way of calculating PTA is recommended.

References

1. Hinton AE, Ramsden RT, Ly RH, et al (1992) Criteria for hearing preservation in acoustic schwannoma surgery: the concept of useful hearing. J Laryngol Otol 106:500–503
2. Gardner G, Robertson JH (1988) Hearing preservation in unilateral acoustic neuroma surgery. Otol Rhinol Laryngol 97:555–566

3. Shelton C (1992) Hearing preservation in acoustic tumor surgery. Otolaryngol Clin N Am 25:609–621
4. Whittaker CK, Luetje CM (1992) Vestibular schwannomas. J Neurosurg 76:897–900
5. Glasscock ME III, Hayes LB, Minor LB, et al (1993) Preservation in hearing in acoustic neuromas. J Neurosurg 78:864–870
6. Sanna M, Karmarkar S, Landolfi M (1995) Hearing preservation in vestibular schwannoma surgery: fact or fantasy? J Laryngol Otol 109:374–380
7. Wade RJ, House WF (1984) Hearing preservation in patients with acoustic neuromas via the middle fossa approach. Otolaryngol Head Neck Surg 92:184–193
8. Committee on Hearing and Equilibrium of the American Academy of Otolaryngology–Head and Neck Surgery (1995) Committee on hearing and equilibrium guidelines for the evaluation of hearing preservation in acoustic neuroma (vestibular schwannoma). Otolaryngol Head Neck Surg 113:179–180
9. Avezaat CJJ, Pauw BKH (1997) Vestibular Schwannomas. Handbook of Clinical Neurology, Vol 24(68): Neuro-Oncology, Part II. Elsevier Science, Amsterdam, pp 421–464
10. Harner SG, Beatty CW, Ebersold MJ (1990) Retrosigmoid removal of acoustic neuroma: experience 1978–1988. Otolaryngol Head Neck Surg 102:40–45
11. Fischer G, Fischer C, Rémond J (1992) Hearing preservation in acoustic neuroma surgery. J Neurosurg 76:910–917
12. Goel A, Sekhar LN, Langheinrich W, et al (1992) Late course of preserved hearing and tinnitus after acoustic neurilemoma surgery. J Neurosurg 77:685–689
13. Nadol JB, Chiong CM, Ojemann RG, et al (1992) Preservation of hearing and facial nerve function in resection of acoustic neuroma. Laryngoscope 102:1153–1158
14. Tatagiba M, Samii M, Matthies M, et al (1992) The significance for postoperative hearing of preserving the labyrinth in acoustic neuroma surgery. J Neurosurg 77:677–684
15. Haines SJ, Levine SC (1993) Intracanalicular acoustic neuroma: early surgery for preservation of hearing. J Neurosurg 79:515–520
16. Sterkers J-M, Morrison GAJ, Sterkers O, et al (1994) Preservation of facial, cochlear, and other nerve functions in acoustic neuroma treatment. Otolaryngol Head Neck Surg 110:146–155
17. Dornhoffer JL, Helms J, Hochmann DH (1995) Hearing preservation in acoustic tumor surgery: results and prognostic factors. Laryngoscope 105:184–187
18. Samii M, Matthies C (1997) Management of 100 vestibular schwannomas (acoustic neuromas): surgical management and results with emphasis on complications and how to avoid them. Neurosurgery 40:11–23
19. Shelton C, House WF (1990) Hearing improvement after acoustic tumor removal. Otolaryngol Head Neck Surg 103:963–965
20. Rosenberg RA, Cohen NL, Ransohoff J (1987) Long-term hearing preservation after acoustic neuroma surgery. Otolaryngol Head Neck Surg 97:270–274
21. Shelton C, Hitselberger WE, House WF, et al (1990) Hearing preservation after acoustic tumor removal: long-term results. Laryngoscope 100:115–119
22. McKenna MJC, Halpin RG, Ojemann JB, et al (1992) Long-term results in patients after surgical removal of acoustic tumors with hearing preservation. Am J Otol 13:134–136
23. Umezu H, Aiba T, Tsuchida S, et al (1996) Early and late postoperative hearing preservation in patients with acoustic neuromas. Neurosurgery 39:267–272

Part 4
Effect of Radiotherapy

Long-Term Follow-up Results with Audiological Assessment After Fractionated Stereotactic Radiotherapy for Vestibular Schwannomas

Yutaka Sawamura, Hiroki Shirato, Touru Sakamoto, Hidefumi Aoyama, Satoshi Fukuda, and Kazuo Miyasaka

Summary. We investigated the appropriate management of patients with vestibular schwannoma treated with fractionated stereotactic radiotherapy (fSRT).

Key words. Vestibular schwannoma, Stereotactic radiation, Radiation therapy, Fractionation, Hearing preservation

One hundred eleven patients with vestibular schwannoma were treated with fSRT at 40–50 Gy in 20–25 fractions over a period of 5–6 weeks. The mean size of the tumors was 15.4 mm (range, 3–40 mm), including 23 tumors over 25 mm. Eighty-four patients (77%) had testable hearing before fSRT. The median follow-up period was 34.7 months. The patients were followed up every 6 months until the fifth year by interviews, neurological and otological examinations, and magnetic resonance imaging. The actuarial 5-year tumor control rate (no tumor growth greater than 2.0 mm and no requirement for salvage resection surgery) was 92% in 64 patients who were followed for more than 24 months (median, 43; range, 24–110). The actuarial 3-year tumor-reduction rate (reduction in tumor size greater than 2.0 mm) was 93%. During the first 2 years after fSRT, some patients had enlargement of the tumor, but most were transient, and only three patients with a progressive tumor underwent salvage tumor removal. Seven patients with progressive hydrocephalus and without any evidence of tumor progression received a Ventriculoperi-

Departments of Neurosurgery, Radiology, and Otolaryngology, Hokkaido University School of Medicine, North 15, West 7, Kita-ku, Sapporo 060-8638, Japan

toneal (V-P) shunt. The actuarial 5-year useful-hearing preservation rate (Gardner-Robertson class I or II) was 73.9% in previously hearing patients. Oral steroid intake was useful for treating hearing deterioration after SRT. None of the 20 patients who were otologically monitored for more than 5 years had further deterioration of hearing. As complications of fSRT, transient facial nerve palsy, trigeminal neuropathy, and dysequilibrium were observed 2.5%, 15.0%, and 17.5% of patients, respectively. No permanent facial palsy occurred.

We concluded that the use of fractionated SRT resulted in an excellent tumor control rate even for relatively large tumors and produced a hearing preservation rate compatible with the best published results of single fraction radiosurgery. Some patients required neurosurgical management for a long time after fSRT or steroid administration; careful long-term observation is, therefore, necessary. This may be also true for radiosurgery.

Gamma Knife Radiosurgery in Vestibular Schwannomas: Clinical and Radiological Impact on the Tumor Course

Massimo Gerosa, Antonio Nicolato, Roberto Foroni, and
Albino Bricolo

Summary. Up to the last decade, therapeutic options for patients with
vestibular schwannomas (VS) were limited to total or subtotal excision or
expectant serial observation. Stereotactic irradiation, and particularly gamma
knife radiosurgery (GKR), have offered an important additional option to the
overall management strategy. Clinical results, in terms both of tumor growth
control (TGC) and of preserved regional cranial nerve function, have increasingly validated this approach in properly selected indications for either
primary or recurrent tumors. Indeed, using current neuroradiological techniques (MRI-CT fusion algorithms) as well as newer radiodosimetry programs and reduced dosages, the reported achievable TGC rate actually
exceeds 90% in mid-term follow-up (5 years), whereas the relevance of radio-
induced cranial neuropathy has been minimized: facial impairment incidence
lower than 3%, with hearing function (Gardner-Robertson [G-R] 1–2) preserved in over 60% of the patients. Our experience, in a series of 170 treated
VS (9.4% NeuroFibromatosis type 2, or NF2) further confirms these data: the
group of evaluable cases (112 patients with over 4 years of mean follow-up)
shows an overall TGC rate of 93%, with an extremely low incidence of facial
impairment (2.7%) and hearing preservation in 66% (G-R 1–2). However,
long-term fullow-up results in large series of patients treated by contemporary GKR techniques are not yet available: with lowering treatment dosages,
surviving tumor cells might sustain a delayed regrowth, eventually decreasing TGC rates. To date, GKR may be advocated for small-to-medium-sized VS,
with negative cranial nerve staging, absent or minimal hearing deficit, and in
several cases with major surgical contraindications or in patients refusing
microsurgery. Furthermore, it is worth stressing that particularly for elderly

Dipartimento di Neurochirurgia, Ospedale di Borgo Trento, Piazzale Stefani 1, 37126
Verona, Italy

patients with larger schwannomas and for NF2 patients, an integrated program including both GKR and microsurgery should always be considered.

Key words. Vestibular schwannoma, Acoustic neuroma, Neurofibromatosis, Radiosurgery, Gamma knife

Introduction

Unilateral vestibular schwannomas (VS) have always been considered typically slow-growing tumors, particularly in elderly patients. Some aspects of the natural course of these lesions have been repeatedly emphasized in the literature: a relatively high incidence (40% to 71%) of "no growth" patterns, even in mid-term follow-up analyses (mean follow-up 26 to 42 months) of selected groups of untreated patients [1–4]; a non-negligible (3%–6%) rate of spontaneous tumor regression [2–4]; and mostly benign behavior of the disease, with very limited anatomical aggressiveness, rare arachnoidal invasiveness, and sluggish neurological impact [3,4]. Therefore, up to the last decade, therapeutic options for these patients were essentially represented by microsurgery or expectant serial observation. However, the unpredictable cell kinetics of these specific oncotypes have been widely documented. The average growth rate in long-term follow-up studies is quite variable, ranging from 0.28 to 6.9 mm/year [1,5–7]. Younger patients and NeuroFibromatosis type 2 (NF2) usually account for faster growth rates [2,6,7]. Furthermore, vascular damage (particularly to the internal auditory artery) may dramatically compromise the neurological picture, even in radiologically quiescent tumors [1,2,7]. In this regard, gamma knife stereotactic radiosurgery (GKR) has offered an important additional option in the overall management strategy, with elective indications in older or medically compromised patients with small-to-medium-sized VS [3,4,6,8–11].

Gamma Knife Stereotactic Radiosurgery

The Focus

Unlike microsurgery, radiosurgery does not remove the neoplastic target but is aimed at dooming the proliferative activity of the tumor. Therefore, the goal of this technique in treating VS is represented by the so-called tumor growth control (TGC), a widely debated concept that entails a peculiar biological rationale and a spectrum of neuroradiological patterns.

The biological rationale is based upon a radio-induced inhibition of tumor cell proliferation by two principal mechanisms (Table 1): direct cytotoxic activity (killing or dooming proliferating cells, apoptotic triggering) and pro-

TABLE 1. Gamma knife radiosurgery in vestibular schwannoma: biological rationale

Cytotoxic effect
    Alpha/beta ratio: slow-growing cells [10,12]
    Time-dose dependency
    Spectrum of variability—in vitro cells surviving 150 Gy dose exposure [12,13]
    Mainly cytoplasmic and membrane lesion ("interphase death") [13]

Vascular lesion
    Concurrent with tissue lesions in the early phase
    Preceding tissue lesions in delayed radionecrotic effects
    Obliterating vasculitis (endothelial proliferation, vessel wall hyalinization) closely
       related to CE (contrast-enhancement) decrease [12–14]

TABLE 2. Gamma knife radiosurgery in vestibular schwannoma: tumor growth control

Permanent in long-term follow-up after higher treatment dosages [15]
Tumor growth control (TGC) rates significantly higher than in comparable groups of
    untreated patients [3,4]
Results confirmed by NF2 "internal control" studies: treated vs. untreated site [6]

gressive radio-obliteration of the tumor vascular supply [10,12,13]. Treatment dosages in these tumors may be relatively low, thereby protecting the brainstem and the adjacent cranial nerves, due to the generally low alpha/beta ratio. However, the radiosensitivity of these oncotypes may be extremely-variable: neuroma cell subsets have been shown to survive in vitro dosages of up to 150 Gy (i.e., 10–12 times the therapeutic edge levels), whereas others may be killed by 8 Gy per single fraction [12,13]. The radiation-induced vascular lesion apparently exploits the well-known differential radiosensitivity of tumor vessels versus normal vessels. The obliteration of the neoplastic vasculature (endothelial proliferation/hyalinization) might explain some late-appearing tumor shrinkage, decreased contrast enhancement, and necrotic evolution [10,13–15].

As a result, treatment effectiveness may be documented by a variety of magnetic resonance pictures, from neoplastic growth arrest to measurable tumor volume reduction [14]. A substantial decrease in size is usually obtained in a percentage of cases: the degree of this shrinkage and the timing of the effect are presumably related to the specific cell kinetics of the treated tumor (to the peculiar "growth fraction" and to the "tumor doubling time," respectively). For instance, in very slow-growing schwannomas, radiosurgical results may become more pronounced even some years after treatment [9–11,14].

There is consistent evidence (Table 2) that radiosurgical TGC is somehow different from the spontaneous "hibernation" of these tumors [3,4,6,9,10] and can be effectively maintained for decades [15].

Indications

Radiosurgical treatment of VS, once anecdotal, has become increasingly frequent during the last decade, according to the impressively growing indications: to date, almost 20 000 VS patients have been treated worldwide by this technique [4,8–11]. However, GKR treatment of VS requires a careful and appropriate staging of eligible patients, including clinical and neuroradiological parameters [4,8,9,16,17] (Table 3). As a consequence, "historical" indications [3,4,6] (small-to-medium-sized VS in patients with unacceptable surgical risks or refusing microsurgery) have gradually been replaced by "elective" indications, as shown in Table 4 [8–11,18,19]. Furthermore, it is well known that microsurgery and stereotactic radiosurgery have been considered mutually exclusive for a long time. The ongoing evaluation process induced by stratification studies will presumably modify the panels of eligibility cri-

TABLE 3. Gamma knife radiosurgery in vestibular schwannoma: preoperative staging

Clinical
    Age
    Risk factor incidence
    Tumor progression rate
    Primary tumor/recurrence
    Solitary schwannoma/NF2
    Cranial nerve functional grading
    Brainstem involvement
    Cerebellar involvement

Neuroradiological
    Tumor volume [4,8–11]
    Critical diameters:
        Midporus transverse diameter (MPTD)
        Pons–petrous distance (PPD) [16–17]
    Regional anatomy (arachnoidal invasiveness, etc.)

TABLE 4. Gamma knife radiosurgery in vestibular schwannoma: elective indications [8–11,18,19]

Small-to-medium (inf. to 30 mm MPTD or 20 mm PPD)
    size VS
Negative cranial nerve staging—minimal hearing deficit
Slow neoplastic progression
Limited brainstem distortion
Highly critical arachnoidal disruption
NF2: VS on the only hearing side

TABLE 5. Vestibular schwannoma: combined surgical/radiosurgical approaches

Larger VS with extremely risky radical resection [4,9–11]
Regrowth or recurrence after either surgical or radiosurgical failure [9–11,18]
NF2: staged procedures [6,9–11,19,20]

teria on both sides, and possibly widen the indications to combined surgical and radiosurgical approaches. The enhancing role of such integrated treatment protocols is summarized in Table 5 [4,8–11,18].

In this regard, NF2 is possibly a convincing instance. Because of the aggressive and invasive behavior of these tumors, their multifocality, and their putatively limited radiosensitivity, combined surgical and radiosurgical or staged GKR procedures have been advocated. The elective GKR targeting should focus on the side either of the growing tumor or of cranial nerve deterioration [6,9–11,19,20].

Results

In the early phase of this experience—approximately from the very beginning in 1969 to the late 1980s—radiosurgical dosages for VS were substantially higher, with marginal doses usually exceeding 16–18 Gy [4,15,21]. The results were certainly rewarding in terms of TGC, with 91% to 93% of the patients showing invariate or decreased tumor volume, and only a minority of cases showing neoplastic progression. Since these series have accumulated the longest follow-up data, it was also possible to substantiate the long-term stability of the cytological dooming. Nevertheless, side effects, particularly as regards cranial neuropathy, were not negligible, with facial involvement reported in up to 17% of cases [3,4,6,15,16] (Table 6).

In the last decade, technical advances have greatly modified both stages of the radiosurgical procedure, i.e., the anatomical localization of the target as well as the radiobiological approach. Neuroradiological upgrades (high-resolution MRI with specific sequences, millimetric slices, multiplanar volume acquisition, CT bone algorithm for cochlear and vestibular structures, use of imaging fusion software, etc.) have dramatically improved the limited, CT-based visualization of the ponto-cerebellar angle, providing an appropriate identification of the regional topography. On the other side, the availability of computerized dosimetry programs (tridimensional matching of the targeted volume, "inverse treatment planning" models, etc.) and the introduction of robotized, automatic positioning systems with submillimetric precision, have allowed multifocal, extremely conformal treatment plans with lower dosages (mostly 12.5–14 Gy to the edge), minimizing undue exposure [8–11].

TABLE 6. Gamma knife radiosurgery in vestibular schwannoma

Historical results [3,4,6,15,16,21]	
TGC	91%–93%
Facial deficit	14%–17%
Trigeminal neuropathy	16%–19%
Hearing preservation (overall)	21%–26%
CSF shunting	5%
Last decade [8–11,19,20]	
TGC	94%–97%
Facial deficit	2%–5%
Trigeminal neuropathy	5%
Hearing preservation (Gardner-Robertson [G-R] 1–2)	45%–71%
CSF shunting	2%

As a result, the slight increase in TGC (94%–97%) has been associated with a drastic reduction of radio-induced sequelae: 95% to 98% facial sparing, exponential drop in trigeminal neuropathy, 45% to 71% hearing preservation on the basis of a Gardner-Robertson (G-R) score of 1 to 2 [8–11,19,20] (Table 6).

Open Questions

Some issues will probably gain further relevance in future comprehensive analyses of GKR results.

Tumor Growth Control

It is generally accepted that dose-volume relations are the major effective limit in obtaining adequate growth control when treating larger tumors. Further obstacles may come from the presence of relevant necrotic-cystic components, even though the real radiobiological impact of such degenerative features is still being debated [17–21]. Moreover, 10 years or longer follow-up in large series of patients treated with contemporary GKR techniques are not yet available. With lowering of treatment dosages, surviving tumor cells might sustain a delayed regrowth, eventually decreasing long-term TGC rates.

Cranial Neuropathy

The mechanism of radio-induced cranial neuropathy is still poorly known. Concomitant damage to axons, myelin, and perineural-pial vessels is possibly involved [12,16,17,21]. Risk factor algorithms should presumably include updated radiobiological parameters such as the average and the integral target dose, the pons-petrous distance for trigeminal involvement, and the mid-porus transverse diameter for facial impairment [9,16–18,21].

Radiation Oncogenesis

The problem has recently been addressed in the literature: two cases of putatively sarcomatous evolution—one GKR-treated VS [22] and one neurofibroma [23]—have been reported. Despite the questionable radiobiological relation and the limited statistical inference (2/20 000 treated cases), the issue certainly deserves increased vigilance.

Cost Analysis

Several health care systems in the world are presently evaluating all the major parameters in regard to cost: cost-effectiveness, cost-benefit, and cost-utility. Radiosurgical equipment is certainly high-priced, and GKR requires prolonged clinical follow-up and repeated, expensive neuroradiological controls. On the other side, a number of parametrized items, i.e., hospitalization time, treatment costs, rehabilitation, time to resuming working activity, and quality of life itself, seem to favor this approach [24]. Recent studies, based on decision-analysis techniques for probabilistic dominance as well as on functional outcome rating scales (FORS), have strongly supported the use of GKR in eligible patients [25,26].

Our Experience

From February 1993 to February 2002, 154 patients with unilateral VS and 12 NF2 patients (16 tumors) were treated by GKR in our department, for a total number of 170 lesions (M/F 88/78; mean age, 59.8 years; range, 19–83; primary tumor/recurrence 88/82). The treatment protocol included clinicoradiological assessment with cranial nerve staging and target localization using combined stereo MRI–stereo CT bone algorithm. The major dose planning parameters were as follows: average tumor volume, 2.6 cc (range, 0.3–12.5); mean peripheral dose, 13.8 Gy (range, 12.0–15.8); average dose, 24.3 Gy (range, 16–30.7); n.isocenters 7.4 [2–19].

To date, 112 patients with a minimum follow-up of 24 months are evaluable. Their mean follow-up time is 49 months (range, 25–102). The radiological and clinical results are briefly summarized in Table 7. The overall TGC was approximately 93%. Treatment failures were observed in a small minority of cases (7.1%). Smaller VS usually showed the best response rates, but unexpectedly pronounced shrinkages were obtained also in rather large, necrotic (Fig. 1) or cystic (Fig. 2) tumors, 14 to 20 months after radiosurgery.

TABLE 7. Our experience: clinical and radiological results (112 patients; mean follow-up, over 4 years)

MRI
  Tumor shrinkage (over 20% tumor volume reduction): 47.3%
  Unchanged tumor volume: 45.6%
  Neoplastic progression: 7.1%

Clinical outcome
  Hearing preservation: 66% (43/65 G-R 1–2)
  Tinnitus attenuation: 55.7% (44/79)
  Vestib. improv. (vertigo-ataxia): 59% (42/71)

Sequelae
  Facial deficit (overall): 2.7%
    Permanent facial paresis: 0.9%
  Trigeminal neuropathy: 7.1%
  Treatment-related vestibulopathy: 1.8%
  Brainstem or cerebellar involvement: 0

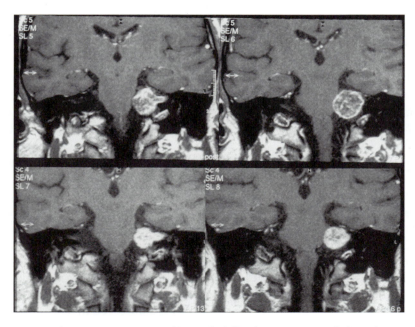

FIG. 1. Large (22 mm pons-petrous distance), diffusely necrotic vestibular schwannoma (VS) (**top**). Pronounced shrinkage 14 months after gamma knife radiosurgery (GKR) (**bottom**). Necrotic and cystic components may sometimes hinder radiosurgical results

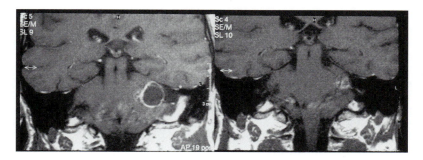

FIG. 2. Typically cystic VS, before (**left**) and 20 months after (**right**) GKR. Another case with drastic tumor regression following radiosurgery

Hearing preservation was possible in 66% of patients with a preoperative G-R of 1–2 (mean follow-up over 4 years). The incidence of adverse effects was negligible: 2.7% facial impairment, with only one case (0.9%) of permanent facial paresis.

Conclusion

Even though the present results seem to validate this approach, it is probably too early for definite conclusions on the future role of the technique in the neurosurgical armamentarium for VS treatment. Newer contributions from so-called outcome analysis will probably become of paramount importance for eligibility criteria protocols as well as for patients' decisions, as recently stressed by the American Acoustic Neuroma Association [25].

References

1. Deen HG, Ebersold MJ, Harner SG, et al (1996) Conservative management of acoustic neuroma: an outcome study. Neurosurgery 39:260–266
2. Bederson JB, von Ammon K, Wichmann WW, et al (1991) Conservative treatment of patients with acoustic tumors. Neurosurgery 28:646–651
3. Lunsford LD, Linskey ME (1992) Stereotactic radiosurgery in the treatment of patients with acoustic tumors. Otolaryngol Head Neck Surg 25:471–491
4. Shetter AG (1997) Gamma knife radiosurgery for the treatment of acoustic neuromas. BNI Q 13:30–36
5. Gardner G, Moretz WH, Robertson JH, et al (1986) Neurosurgical management of small and intracanalicular acoustic tumors. Otolaryngol Head Neck Surg 94:328–333
6. Linskey ME, Lunsford LD, Flickinger JC (1992) Tumor control after stereotactic radiosurgery in neurofibromatosis patients with bilateral acoustic tumors. Neurosurgery 31:829–839
7. Nedzelski JM, Schessel DA, Pfeiderer A, et al (1992) The natural history of acoustic neuromas and its role in non invasive management. In: Tos M, Thomsen J (eds)

Acoustic neuroma: proceedings of the first international conference on acoustic neuromas. Copenhagen, Denmark, August 25–29, 1991. Kugler, Amsterdam, pp 149–158

8. Bertalanffy A, Dietrich W, Aichholzer M, et al (2001) Gamma knife radiosurgery of acoustic neurinomas. Acta Neurochir (Wien) 143:689–695

9. Flickinger JC, Kondziolka D, Niranjan A, et al (2001) Results of acoustic neuroma radiosurgery: an analysis of 5 years' experence using current methods. J Neurosurg 94: 1–6

10. Linskey ME (2000) Stereotactic radiosurgery versus stereotactic radiotherapy for patients with vestibular schwannoma: a Leksell Gamma Knife Society 2000 debate. J Neurosurg 93:90–95

11. Kondziolka D, Lunsford LD, Flickinger JC (2000) Gamma knife radiosurgery for vestibular schwannomas. Neurosurg Clin North Am 11:651–658

12. Linskey ME, Martinez AS, Kondziolka D, et al (1993) The radiobiology of human acoustic schwannoma xenografts after stereotactic radiosurgery, evaluated in the subrenal capsule of athymic mice. J Neurosurg 78:645–653

13. Anniko M, Arndt J, Norèn G (1981) The human acoustic neuroma in organ culture. Acta Otolaryngol 91:223–225

14. Linskey ME, Lunsford LD, Flickinger JC (1991) Neuroimaging of acoustic nerve tumors after stereotaxic radiosurgery. AJNR 12:1165–1175

15. Norèn G, Hirsch A, Mosskin M (1993) Long term efficacy of gamma knife radiosurgery in vestibular schwannomas (abstract). Acta Neurochir (Wien) 122:164

16. Linskey ME, Flickinger JC, Lunsford LD (1993) Cranial nerve length predicts the risk of delayed facial and trigeminal neuropathies after acoustic tumor, stereotactic radiosurgery. Int J Radiat Oncol Biol Phys 25:227–233

17. Foote KD, Friedman WA, Buatti JM, et al (2001) Analysis of risk factors associated with radiosurgery for vestibular schwannoma. J Neurosurg 95:440–449

18. Pollock BE, Lunsford LD, Kondziolka D, et al (1998) Vestibular schwannoma management. Part II—Failed radiosurgery and the role of delayed microsurgery. J Neurosurg 89:949–955

19. Roche PH, Regis J, Pellet W, et al (2000) Neurofibromatosis type 2—preliminary results of gamma knife radiosurgery of vestibular schwannomas. Neurochirurgie 46:339–353

20. Kida Y, Kobayashi T, Tanaka T, et al (2000) Radiosurgery for bilateral neurinomas associated with neurofibromatosis type 2. Surg Neurol 53:383–389

21. Noren G (1998) Long term complication following gamma knife radiosurgery of vestibular schwannomas. Stereotact Funct Neurosurg 70 (suppl 1):65–73

22. Hanabusa K, Marikawa A, Murata T, et al (2001) Acoustic neuroma with malignant transformation. J Neurosurg 95:518–521

23. Thomsen J, Mirz F, Wetke R (2000) Intracranial sarcoma in a patient with neurofibromatosis type-2 treated with gamma knife radiosurgery for vestibular schwannoma. Am J Otol 21:364–370

24. Van Roijen N, Nijs HGT, Avezaat CJJ, et al (1997) Costs and effects of microsurgery versus radiosurgery in treating acoustic neuroma. Acta Neurochir (Wien) 139:942–948

25. Hudgins WR (1994) Patients' attitude about outcomes and the role of gamma knife radiosurgery in the treatment of vestibular schwannomas. Neurosurgery 34:459–465

26. Pollock BE, Lunsford LD, Kondziolka D, et al (1995) Outcome analysis of acoustic neuroma management: a comparison of microsugery and stereotactic radiosurgery. Neurosurgery 36:215–229

Part 5
Neurological Symptoms and Other Related Items

Functional Staging of Acoustic Neuromas

ALEXIS BOZORG GRAYELI[1], MICHEL KALAMARIDES[2], DIDIER BOUCCARA[1], ALAIN REY[2], and OLIVIER STERKERS[1]

Summary. Facial function and hearing preservation are the two main challenges in acoustic neuroma surgery. A retrospective study of 441 patients [192 males and 249 females; mean age; 60 years (range, 16–79)] who were operated on for a unilateral acoustic neuroma was undertaken. The mean diameter of the tumors was $26 \pm 0.6\,mm$. One hundred four patients (14%) were operated on through conservative approaches (middle cranial fossa and retrosigmoid) and 335 (76%) through the translabyrinthine route. A cutoff value for the tumor diameter in the cerebellopontine angle (CPA) was observed at 15 mm in terms of postoperative facial and hearing function. Among lesions operated on through conservative approaches, hearing preservation was obtained in 63% and 14% of patients with tumors measuring less than 15 mm and between 16 and 20 mm in the CPA, respectively. The proportion of good facial function 1 year after surgery with tumors between 11 and 15 mm and between 16 and 20 mm was 91% and 73%, respectively. In conclusion, a classification is proposed subdividing the lesions as follows: stage 1, intracanalicular; stage 2, less than 15 mm in the CPA; stage 3, 15–30 mm in the CPA; stage 4, more than 30 mm in the CPA. This classification appears to be well correlated to facial function prognosis and the possibility of hearing function preservation.

Keywords. Surgery, Facial function, Hearing preservation, Prognosis, Vestibular schwannoma

[1]Department of Otolaryngology and INSERM E0112, [2]Department of Neurosurgery, Hôpital Beaujon, 100 Boulevard du Général Leclerc, 92118 Clichy Cedex, France

Introduction

Many classifications have been proposed for acoustic neuromas based on pre-operative imaging data. The multitude of classifications hampers the comparison of postoperative functional results, and authors should tend toward a unique system for reporting clinical data on acoustic neuromas. A classification should meet two objectives, which are simplicity and significance in terms of prognosis.

The aim of this study was to compare two classifications in terms of pre-operative and postoperative clinical, audiometric, and imaging data and to evaluate the significance of these classifications in terms of functional prognosis.

Material and Methods

A retrospective study was undertaken including 441 patients operated on for a vestibular schwannoma between 1987 and 2001. The population comprised 192 males and 249 females. The mean age was 60 years, ranging between 16 and 79 years. All patients underwent preoperative clinical evaluation, audiometry, video-nystagmography, auditory evoked potentials, magnetic resonance imaging (MRI), and computed tomography (CT) scanning. Patients were operated on through a translabyrinthine (TL) route in 335 cases (76%), a retrosigmoid (RS) route in 60 cases (14%), and a middle cranial fossa (MCF) approach in 46 patients (10%). The mean postoperative follow-up period was 19 months, ranging from 12 to 108 months. Clinical data were obtained from medical files concerning preoperative neurological deficits, audiovestibular status, MRI, postoperative deficits, complications, quality of resection, and recurrence. The House and Brackmann classification was used for assessment of facial function [1]. A good facial function was defined as grades 1 and 2. The American Academy of Otolaryngology–Head and Neck Surgery (AAO–HNS) classification was employed for hearing function evaluation. Useful hearing was considered as classes A and B [2].

Tumor size was expressed according to two different classifications:

Classification 1:
    Stage 1: intracanalicular
    Stage 2: lesions ≤2 cm in the cerebellopontine angle (CPA)
    Stage 3: lesions ≤4 cm and >2 cm in the CPA
    Stage 4: lesions >4 cm in the CPA
Classification 2:
    Stage 1: intracanalicular
    Stage 2: lesions ≤1.5 cm in the CPA
    Stage 3: lesions ≤3 cm and >1.5 cm in the CPA
    Stage 4: lesions >3 cm in the CPA

Results

Preoperative Deficits

Preoperative facial function was evaluated as grade 1 in 388 cases (88%), as grade 2 in 52 cases (11%), as grade 3, 4, and 5 in 1 case each, and as grade 6 in 2 cases. Preoperative hearing function was assessed as class A in 117 cases (27%), as class B in 110 cases (25%), as class C in 133 cases (30%), and as class D in 81 cases (18%).

Preoperative Imaging

The greatest tumor diameter in the CPA on axial views of preoperative imaging is represented in Fig. 1. The majority of the lesions (334 lesions, 76%) measured between 1 and 30 mm in the CPA. According to tumor size classification 1, 36 (9%) stage 1, 239 (49%) stage 2, 156 (33%) stage 3, and 11 (9%) stage 4 lesions could be distinguished. According to tumor size classification 2, 36 (9%) stage 1, 184 (41%) stage 2, 160 (36%) stage 3, and 61 (14%) stage 4 lesions were noted.

In both classifications, the relationship between the frequency of preoperative facial paresis and tumor size could be evidenced (data not shown). Similarly, both classifications showed a significant decrease of the proportion of useful hearing with increasing tumor size (data not shown).

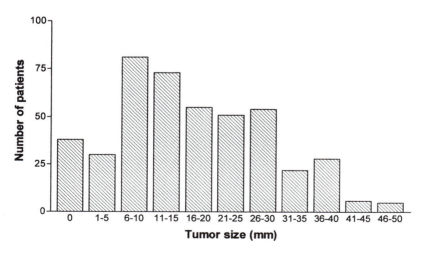

FIG. 1. Relative frequency of cases as a function of tumor size. Tumor size was assessed as the greatest diameter of the lesion on axial views of preoperative MRI ($n = 441$)

Postoperative Results

Facial Function

Data on postoperative facial function were obtained in 365 cases. A grade 1 facial function was reported in 207 cases (57%), grade 2 in 62 (17%), grade 3 in 42 (12%), grade 4 in 26 (7%), grade 5 in 19 (5%), and grade 6 in 9 cases (2%). No differences were observed between RS, MCF, and TL routes for good postoperative facial function in lesions measuring less than 20 mm in the CPA (97%, 84%, and 90% of grades 1 and 2, $n = 60$, 46, and 97, respectively; Fischer's test).

The proportion of good facial function (grades 1 and 2) as a function of tumor size is represented in Fig. 2. A tumor diameter of 15 mm appeared to be a cutoff value for facial function prognosis because a decrease of proportion of good facial function was observed between tumor subgroups measuring 11–15 mm and 16–20 mm (91% versus 73%, $n = 60$ and 46, respectively; $P = 0.02$, Fischer's test).

Hearing Function

The RS and MCF routes were employed for hearing preservation in 89 patients with preoperative useful hearing (classes A and B) and lesions measuring less than 20 mm in the CPA. These approaches were also used in 17 patients with preoperative classes C and D. Among patients with useful preoperative hearing, postoperative hearing was evaluated as class A in 13 cases (15%), as class B in 24 cases (27%), as class C in 19 cases (19%), and as class D in 35

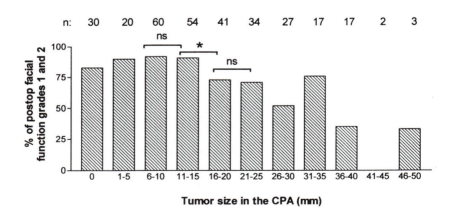

FIG. 2. Percentage of good postoperative facial function (grades 1 and 2) as a function of tumor size in patients with normal preoperative facial function. Tumor size was assessed as the greatest diameter of the lesion on axial views of preoperative MRI. *CPA*, cerebellopontine angle. *$P < 0.05$, *ns* (nonsignificant), Fischer's test

FIG. 3. Percentage of postoperative hearing function preservation as a function of tumor size. Hearing preservation was defined by hearing function of class A, B, or C (AAO-HNS classification) 1 year after surgery. *$P < 0.05$, Fischer's test

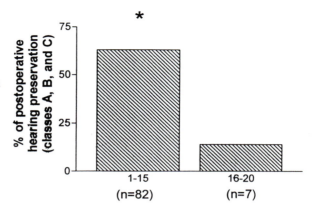

Tumor size in the CPA (mm)

cases (39%). When expressed as a function of tumor size, the hearing preservation results showed that the proportion of cases with preserved hearing decreased significantly for tumors measuring more than 15 mm (Fig. 3).

Discussion

Many classifications have been proposed for acoustic neuromas based on their size, as determined by preoperative imaging [3,4]. Comparison of classifications 1 and 2 showed that the discrimination between stages 2 and 3 in terms of postoperative auditory and facial function by classification 2, was powerful. Furthermore, classifications 1 and 2 did not show obvious differences in terms of preoperative facial and hearing function. The use of classification 2 is justified by a better prognostic value concerning postoperative facial function and hearing preservation.

Measurement of tumor diameter on MRI axial views appears to be a simple method that has prognosis significance in terms of postoperative functional results. The measurement of tumor volume on MRI appears to be important in patients who are conservatively managed by the watch-and-scan policy [5]. Nevertheless, routine application of this method is now limited to a few centers.

References

1. House JW, Brackmann DE (1985) Facial nerve grading system. Otolaryngol Head Neck Surg 3:184–193
2. Committee on Hearing and Equilibrium (1995) Guidelines for the evaluation of hearing preservation in acoustic neuroma (vestibular schwannoma). Otolaryngol Head Neck Surg 113:179–180

3. Tos M, Thomsen J (1992) Synopsis on disagreement in measuring tumor size at the Copenhagen acoustic neuroma conference. In: Tos M, Thomsen J (eds) Acoustic neuroma. Kugler, Amsterdam, pp 975–978
4. Pulec JL, House WF, Britton WH (1971) A system of management of acoustic neuroma based on 364 cases. Trans Am Acad Ophthalmol Oto-Laryngol 75:48–55
5. Charabi S, Thomsen J, Mantoni M, et al. (1995) Acoustic neuroma: growth and surgical and nonsurgical consequences of the wait and see policy. Otolaryngol Head Neck Surg 113:5–14

Evaluation of Tinnitus Before and After Microsurgical Resection of Acoustic Tumors

Tomio Sasaki, Katsushige Watanabe, Takashi Watanabe, and Nobuto Saito

Before treating patients with acoustic tumors, doctors must take into account the benefits and risks resulting from the treatment. Information regarding risks includes the associated mortality and morbidity, such as cerebellar dysfunction, facial nerve palsy, and hearing loss.

The effects of the treatment on the tinnitus are sometimes ignored and are not explained to the patient. Moreover, there have been few reports on the effects of the treatment on tinnitus. More information should be collected.

We evaluated the effects of microsurgical resection of acoustic tumors on tinnitus in 149 patients. Altogether, 109 (73.2%) of the 149 patients complained of tinnitus before the operation. Among them, the tinnitus disappeared after the operation in 25 patients (22.9%), persisted but decreased in 37 (33.9%), did not change in 32 (29.4%), and increased in 15 (13.8%). Among the 40 patients without tinnitus before the operation, only 2 complained of tinnitus after the operation.

We propose a new grading system for evaluating tinnitus more accurately. Tinnitus before treatment could be graded into four groups: (1) none; (2) slight (small amount of noise inoffensive to the ear during daily life); (3) moderate (noise offensive to the ear during daily life); and (4) severe (noise that disturbs sleeping). Tinnitus after treatment was graded into four groups considering the treatment's effect: (1) none; (2) persisting but decreased; (3) persisting the same as before; and (4) persisting and increased.

Department of Neurosurgery, Gunma University, School of Medicine, Gunma, Japan

Indices of Facial Features Obtained from Contour Extraction with Image Processing and Its Application to Objective Estimation of Facial Palsy

Toshiyuki Tanaka[1], Shohei Orukawa[1], Noriyuki Yoshida[1], and Takanobu Kunihiro[2]

Summary. This chapter deals with a method for evaluating facial nerve palsy using the shapes of the lips and eyes. It is difficult to establish the condition of the patient's recovery using previous evaluation methods. In recent years, recognition technology and synthesis technology of the human face have been studied by many researchers, mainly from the viewpoint of applying engineering principles to a communication media–human interface. We have applied a recognition method of the human face to an evaluation of facial nerve palsy. We obtained contours of the lips and eyes using image processing by utilizing color information from the digital image. Next, we tracked the changing contours during lip motion, and defined seven indices in our proposed method for grading the palsy. Finally, we evaluated the validity of this method in healthy persons and palsy subjects. The seven indices were modified so the values were 0 for healthy persons. As the palsy became more severe, the indices increased. Differences between the grades of facial palsy appeared as differences in our proposed indices. Good evaluation results were obtained when this method was used for palsy subjects. It thus seems that this method could be effectively utilized to observe the recovery from palsy.

Key words. Facial nerve palsy, Evaluation, Image processing, Contour extraction, Indices of facial palsy

[1] Department of Applied Physics and Physico-Informatics, Faculty of Science and Technology, Keio University, 3-14-1 Hiyoshi, Kohoku-ku, Yokohama 223-8522, Japan
[2] Department of Otorhinolaryngology, School of Medicine, Keio University, Shinjuku-ku, Tokyo 160-8582, Japan

Introduction

In Japan the 40-points method and the facial nerve grading system are generally used to evaluate facial palsy. Based on facial motion, they do not require special devices and are easily performed by simple inspection. In countries other than Japan, the House-Brackmann method [1] is widely used, where doctors evaluate facial palsy based on facial motions. These methods have limited precision, however, as the clinical result is influenced by the subjectivity of the doctor; but even objectivity and reproducibility would not be enough. It is difficult to determine the amount of recovery from these evaluation methods. Various attempts [2–4] have been made to solve these problems, such as developing methods with more objectivity and reproducibility, but they have not yet been widely applied.

In recent years, recognition technology [5–11] and synthesis technology of the human face have been studied mainly from the viewpoint of applying a communication media–human interface using engineering principles. With such applications, image processing is used to analyze a facial expression. Since the advent of computers, analyzing facial expression with high-grade image-processing technology has become easy. Image processors such as video cameras and digital cameras and image scanners, have been developed and are inexpensive. Interest in handling facial information has increased in the fields of psychology, anthropology, dentistry, and makeup and the arts, among others.

Evaluation of facial palsy with image-processing technology has been attempted in the medical field. One such method measures the postions of several marks on the face; another uses moiré stripes [4]. A number of researchers in Japan have attempted to use some of these methods, but they are not widely used for diagnostic purposes. We propose a method for evaluating facial palsy with image processing, using the shape of the contours of the lips and eyes.

Materials and Methods

In many cases, facial nerve symptoms appear in either the left side or the right side of the face. Therefore, by noting the symmetry of the face we can expect that the precise contours of the lips and eyes can be helpful when applied to the evaluation. In this study we developed an accurate contour extraction system and utilized it for objectively diagnosing facial palsy.

Contour Extraction of the Lips and Eyes

First, data were extracted concerning contours of the lips and eyes. The whole facial region was mapped using color information on Japanese subjects. The lips are located in the lower, central area of the face, and the eyes are located in the upper left and upper right regions of the face. The lips and eyes were examined for exact color information. Most procedures are done automatically using image processing.

Palsy Indices Obtained by Shapes of Lips and Eyes

We propose seven indices for evaluating facial palsy. The reference point of the face (center) is determined as shown in Fig. 1 before the indices are computed. The central line is a line going through the central point of the face.

Ratio of the Area of Lip Regions (Affected Side/Healthy Side). The first index is the ratio of the area of the lip region. The affected and healthy sides are separated by the central line of the face, as shown in Fig. 2.

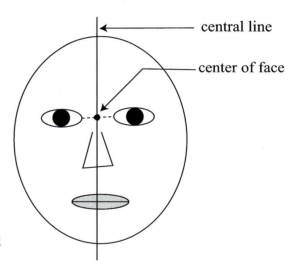

FIG. 1. Center of the face and the central line

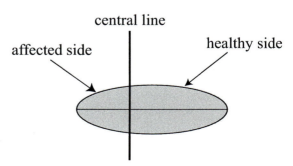

FIG. 2. Affected side and healthy side in the mouth area

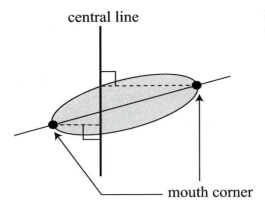

central line

FIG. 3. Mouth corner and the position of the mouth corners

mouth corner

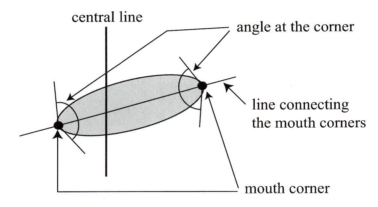

central line

angle at the corner

line connecting the mouth corners

mouth corner

FIG. 4. Angle at the corner and line connecting the mouth corners

$$\text{Index } 1 = \left|1 - \frac{\text{area of affected lip region}}{\text{area of healthy lip region}}\right| \tag{1}$$

Ratio of the Position of the Mouth corners. The second index requires mouth corners. Mouth corners are the left and right edges of the mouth that were determined using image processing, as shown in Fig. 3.

$$\text{Index } 2 = \left|1 - \frac{\text{x coordinate of diseased angle of the mouth}}{\text{x coordinate of healthy angle of the mouth}}\right| \tag{2}$$

Ratio of Angles at the Corners of the Mouth. The third index requires the angle at the corner of the mouth. We define this angle as shown in Fig. 4.

FIG. 5. Distance between the center of the lip region and the central line

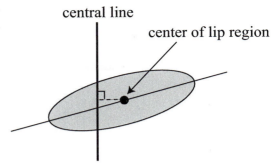

central line

center of lip region

$$\text{Index } 3 = \left| 1 - \frac{\text{diseased angle of mouth}}{\text{healthy angle of mouth}} \right| \tag{3}$$

Absolute Value of the Slope of the Line Connecting the Mouth Corners. The fourth index requires the line connecting the mouth corners, which is defined in Fig. 4.

Distance Between Center of Lip Region and Central Line of the Face. The fifth index is the distance between the center of the lip region and the central line. The distance is defined in Fig. 5.

Index of the Circle of the Lip Contours. The sixth index is the grade of the circle of the lip. The grade of the circle is defined by the following equation.

$$e = 4\pi \frac{\text{area of lip region}}{(\text{perimeter of lip region})^2} \tag{4}$$

This index shows how circular the shape of the lip region is. If the shape is perfectly circular, the index is 1. The index of the circle is used to assess facial palsy only during the whistle motion.

Ratio of the Area of the Closed Eye to the Area of the Eye at Rest. The seventh index is the ratio of the area of the eye region at closing to that at rest.

$$\text{Index } 7 = \frac{\text{eye's area at closing}}{\text{eye's area at rest}} \tag{5}$$

The above indices are modified so the values are approximately 1.0 for healthy persons. We prepared graphs of changes in the above indices, which indicate recovery from facial palsy.

Results

The results of image processing for facial nerve palsy are as follows. The initial image was made from a photograph obtained under room lights with a black screen behind the subject. The image was converted to a digital image of 640

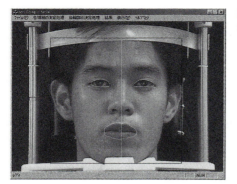

FIG. 6. Contour extraction of lip and eyes at rest

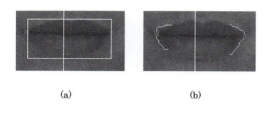

(a)   (b)

FIG. 7. **a** Mouth corners. **b** Contour near the mouth corner

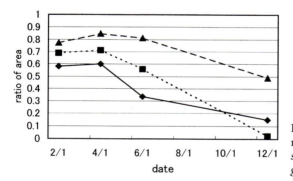

FIG. 8. Ratio of the area of the lip regions. *Diamonds*, face at rest; *squares*, grinning position; *triangles*, whistling position

× 480 pixels. After the facial region was recorded from the initial image, the lip and eye regions were determined from the facial image, as shown in Fig. 6. The contours of the lips and eyes are superimposed on the initial image in Fig. 6. We next determined the mouth corners (Fig. 7a) and the angles at the mouth corners (Fig. 7b). The expressions at rest, grinning, and whistling are used for the facial expression with this method. The time courses of the seven proposed indices are shown in Figs. 8–14. Figure 8 shows the time course of the ratio of the areas of the lips, Fig. 9 the time course of the ratio of the position of the mouth corners, Fig. 10 the time course of the ratio of the angle at the corners of the mouth, Fig. 11 the time course of the absolute value of the

FIG. 9. Ratio of the position of the mouth corner. For definition of symbols, see Fig. 8

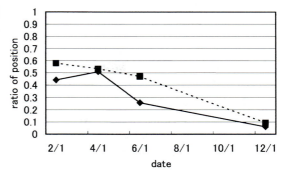

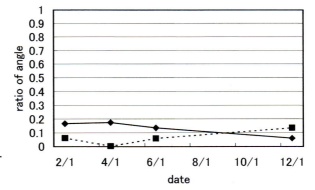

FIG. 10. Ratio of the angle at the corners of the mouth. For definition of symbols, see Fig. 8

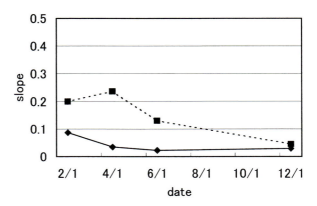

FIG. 11. Absolute value of the slope of the line connecting the mouth corners. For definition of symbols, see Fig. 8

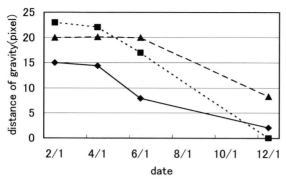

FIG. 12. Distance between the center of the lip region and the central line fo the facial region. For definition of symbols, see Fig. 8

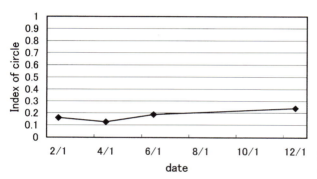

FIG. 13. Index of the circle of the lip region

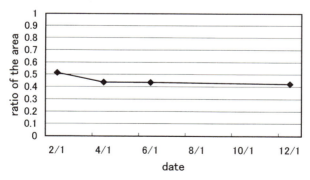

FIG. 14. Ratio of the area of the closed eye to the area of the eye at rest

slope of the line connecting the mouth corners, Fig. 12 the time course of the distance between the center of the lips and the central line of the face, Fig. 13 the time course of the index of the circle of the lips contour, and Fig. 14 the time course of the ratio of the areas of the closed eyes to the eyes at rest.

Discussion

Our proposed indices are modified so they have a value near 0 for healthy persons and a higher value for facial palsy subjects. Figures 8 to 14 show the time courses for facial palsy in the same person from February 1 to December 1. During this period the subject was diagnosed four times and rehabilitiation was undertaken. Figures 8, 9, and 12 obviously show that the values of the indices decreased to 0 during the time they were determined. The physician in charge had assessed by another method that this palsy subject was gradually recovering from the facial palsy. The indices described herein are thus valid for assessing facial palsy. Figure 11 shows that this index is not sufficient for the eye at rest, although the index is good for the grinning motion. Figures 10, 13, and 14 indicate that these indices are not enough to assess facial nerve palsy in terms of the eye at rest or with grinning motions.

We confirmed the validity of our proposed method by applying it to several palsy subjects, where it gave good results. Moreover, it was confirmed that the objectivity and reproducibility of the system are sufficient for assessing facial nerve palsy.

Conclusions

This study dealt with estimating the severity of facial nerve palsy using contour extraction by luminance inphase quadratire (YIQ) and hue value chroma (HVC) bases. The YIQ base is obtained by converting red green blue (RGB). The HVC base is uniform color space. We proposed a regional decision method for the lips and eyes and utilized it for determining their contours. It was possible to determine the exact lip contour when the mouth was opened, whereas it was difficult using other, previous methods. Even though the proposed method is semiautomated, it is easy to use. The results of the contour determination were applied to assess facial nerve palsy. We used the system to follow the time course of recovery from facial nerve palsy. To assess facial palsy, we propose seven indices using the shapes of the lips and eyes. The proposed indices were modified so they were near 0 for healthy persons and were higher for facial palsy subjects. The time courses of three indices showed good results in regard to the palsy. One index showed good results for the grinning motion but was not sufficiently accurate when the face was at rest. The remaining three indices were not accurate enough for the assessment of facial palsy.

We concluded that the "ratio of the area of the lip region," the "ratio of the position of the mouth corners," the "distance between the center of the lip region and the central line of the facial region" indices are good for assessing facial palsy. Thus, we concluded that our proposed method is valid for digitizing the palsy grade and for assessing facial nerve palsy.

Acknowledgment. The authors thank Haruyuki Minamitani and Teruo Miyashita of the Faculty of Science and Technology, Keio University, for suggesting this topic.

References

1. House JW (1983) Facial nerve grading systems. Laryngoscope 93:1056–1069
2. Scriba H, Stoeckli SJ, Veraguth D, Pollak A, Fisch U (1999) Objective evaluation of normal facial function. Ann Otol Rhinol Laryngol 108:641–644
3. Tiffany D, Helling J, Neely G (1997) Validation of objective measures for facial palsy. Laryngoscope 107:1345–1349
4. Yuen K, Kawakami S, Ogawara T, Inokuchi I, Maeta M, Masuda Y (1994) Evaluation of facial palsy by Moiré topography. Eur Arch Otorhinolaryngol [Suppl]:541–544
5. Kass M, Witkin A, Terzopoulos D (1987) Snake: active Contour models. Int J Comput Vis 1(4):321–331
6. Mirhosseini AR, Chen C, Lam KM, Yan H (1997) A Hierarchical and adaptive deformable model for mouth boundary detection. In: 1997 International Conference on Image Processing 2:756–759
7. Ebine H, Nakamura O (1999) The Recognition of facial expressions based on production system. CJECE 24(3):99–107
8. Essa IA, Pantland AP (1995) Facial expression recognition using a dynamic model and motion energy. In: IEEE Proceedings of the 5th International Conference on Computer Vision, pp 360–367
9. Yuille AL, Hallinan PW, Cohen DS (1992) Feature extraction from faces using deformable templates. Int J Comput Vis 8(2):99–111
10. Lanites A, Taylor CJ, Cootes TF (1997) Automatic interpretation and coding of images using flexible model. IEEE Trans Patt Anal Math Intell 19:743–756
11. Harashima H, Aizawa K, Saito T (1989) Model-based analysis synthesis coding of videotelephone images: conception and basic study of intelligent image coding. IEICE Trans E72:452–459
12. Newhall SM, Nickerson D, Judd DB (1943) Final report of the O.S.A subcommittee on the spacing of the Munsell colors. J Opt Soc Am 33:385–418

Part 6
Summaries of Meeting Sessions

Session I: Reporting the Size of Vestibular Schwannomas

Mirko Tos[1], Sho Hashimoto[2], and Jin Kanzaki[3]

Key words. Vestibular schwannoma (size, classification), Acoustic neuroma (size, classification)

Introduction

Forty otoneurosurgeons, neurosurgeons, and neuroradiologists met at the consensus meeting on reporting systems for vestibular schwannomas in November 2001 at Keio University in Tokyo. They arrived at the following agreement for reporting the size of vestibular schwannomas.

1. We need a uniform classification for reporting the size of vestibular schwannomas.
2. Such a classification should be used by all professionals involved in the diagnosis and management of vestibular schwannomas (i.e., general physicians, audiologists, otorhinolaryngologists, neurologists, neurosurgeons, and neuroradiologists).
3. The classification system should be based on measurements only.
4. It should be applied before surgery, that is, based on preoperative computed tomography (CT) or magnetic resonance imaging (MRI) scans.
5. It should be easy to learn and use.
6. It should be easy to imagine; therefore, linear sizes in millimeters should be used instead of volumetric or planimetric measurements.

[1] ENT Department, Gentofte Hospital, University of Copenhagen, DK-2900 Hellerup, Denmark
[2] Department of Otolaryngology, Tohoku University, Graduate School of Medicine, Miyagi, Japan
[3] Department of Otolaryngology, School of Medicine, Keio University, Tokyo, Japan

7. It should be understandable to patients when the tumor is followed by observing its growth with a "wait and see" regimen.
8. It should clearly distinguish between the intracanalicular or intrameatal and extrameatal portion of the tumor.
9. If the intracanalicular portion of the tumor is limited, with no extension out of the porus, the term intrameatal should be used. The size of the extrameatal part of such a tumor is then reported to be 0mm.

Based on the largest extrameatal diameter, the following classification is recommended:

Intrameatal tumor
Grade 1   small   (1–10 mm extrameatal)
Grade 2   medium   (11–20 mm)
Grade 3   moderately large (21–30 mm)
Grade 4   Large   (31–40 mm)
Grade 5   Giant   (>40 mm)

It should be noted if the fundus is empty. The size of the intrameatal tumor can be noted separately by its length and width. (e.g., 5 × 10 mm, but the size of the intrameatal portion should not be added to the extrameatal tumor size. It should also be noted if the tumor is cystic.

Session I: Reporting System for the Size and Site of Residual Vestibular Schwannomas

Mirko Tos[1], Sho Hashimoto[2], and Jin Kanzaki[3]

Key words. Vestibular schwannoma (residual size, residuum classification), Acoustic neuroma (residual size, residuum classification)

Introduction

Even though surgeons prefer to remove a tumor totally, there are situations where a piece of the tumor must be left in place deliberately to save the facial nerve or to avoid damage to vital structures of the brain stem or the anterior inferior cerebellar artery (AICA): This is particularly true today, with "wait and scan" management and radiotherapy for vestibular schwannomas having become accepted as treatment for small and medium-sized tumors; in such cases the growth of the tumor is followed by regularly repeated CT or MRI scanning at various intervals. Postsurgical residual tumor should be managed in the same way.

At the consensus meeting on reporting systems for vestibular schwannomas at Keio University in Tokyo in 2001, forty otoneurosurgeons, neurosurgeons, and neuroradiologists agreed on the following classification for reporting the size and site of residual tumor as well as its regular follow-up.

---

[1] ENT Department, Gentofte University Hospital, University of Copenhagen, DK-2900 Hellerup, Denmark
[2] Deptartment of Otolaryngology, Tohoku University, Graduate School of Medicine, Miyagi, Japan
[3] Deptartment of Otolaryngology, School of Medicine, Keio University, Tokyo, Japan

Classifying Tumor Removal

Total removal
Near-total removal: up to 2% of the tumor is left
Partial removal: up to 5% of the tumor is left
Subtotal removal: more than 5% of the tumor is left

Objective Measurements of Peroperative Size and Site of Residual Tumor

The size of the residual tumor is described in its two perpendicular diameters (in millimeters). It may be found (1) within the meatus; (2) outside meatus along the nerves; or (3) at the brain stem or cerebellum.

Residual Tumor Followed by Repeated CT or MRI Scanning

The timing of CT or MRI scans is as follows: (1) first time within 6 months; (2) second time within 1 year (depending on size); and (3) a CT or MRI scan each year, depending on the size of the lesion.

To follow and classify tumor growth after the first CT or MRI scan, the accepted classification based on the largest extrameatal diameter, is applied. This is:

Intrameatal tumor
Grade 1:   small (1–10 mm)
Grade 2:   medium (11–20 mm)
Grade 3:   moderately large (21–30 mm)
Grade 4:   large (31–40 mm)
Grade 5:   giant (>40 mm)

Session II: Grading Systems for Facial Nerve Function

David A. Moffat[1] and Naoaki Yanagihara[2]

Summary. Consensus has yet to be reached on a system of grading facial nerve function which is accurate and as objective as possible with acceptably small interobserver variability. It is only when this classification has been agreed that meaningful comparison of surgical outcome between various surgical units can be made. The system must reflect the patient's quality of life particularly with regard to the eye and therefore include a grading of synkinesis including hemifacial spasm and also a means of recording nervus intermedius function.

Key words. Vestibular schwannoma, Surgery, Facial nerve function, House-Brackmann classification, Moffat, Modification

Facial Nerve Function

The House-Brackmann (HB) grading system for facial nerve function was an advance and has been successfully used throughout the world for a number of years. It has enabled a meaningful comparison of facial nerve outcome after vestibular schwannoma surgery to be made between various surgical units. The interobserver variability has been found to be small and it is therefore a reliable measure. The well-recognized problem with this classification, however, has been House Grade III. This grade of function has generally been regarded by surgeons as a satisfactory facial nerve outcome and indeed most

---

[1] Department of Otoneurological and Skull Base Surgery, Addenbrooke's Hospital, Cambridge University, Teaching Hospital Trust, Cambridge, UK
[2] Department of Otolaryngology, Takanoko Hospital, Ehime, Japan

TABLE 1. Facial nerve grading system

Grade		Description
I		Normal facial function in all areas
II		
	Gross	Slight weakness noticeable on close inspection
	Synkinesis[a]	Very slight; noticeable on close inspection when the mouth is protruded forcibly
	At rest	Normal symmetry and tone
	Motions	Forehead: moderate to good function
		Eye: complete closure with minimal effort
		Mouth: slight asymmetry
IIIA		
	Gross	Obvious but not disfiguring difference between the two sides
	Synkinesis[a]	Slight; noticeable but not complete when the mouth is protruded forcibly; some contracture and/or hemifacial spasm may be present
	At rest	Normal symmetry and tone
	Motion	Forehead: slight to moderate movements
		Eye: complete closure with effort; eye comfortable and in good condition with or without lubricants
		Mouth: weak with maximum effort
IIIB		
	Gross	Obvious but not disfiguring difference between the two sides.
	Synkinesis[a]	Moderate; eye closes completely when the mouth is protruded forcibly; some contracture and/or hemifacial spasm may be present
	At rest	Normal symmetry and tone
	Motion	Forehead: slight to moderate movement
		Eye: complete closure with effort; eye dry and uncomfortable with evidence of exposure keratitis requiring lubricants and possibly tarsorrhaphy
		Mouth: weak with maximum effort
IV		
	Gross	Obvious weakness and disfiguring asymmetry
	Synkinesis[a]	Severe; apparent mass motion while speaking
	At rest	Normal symmetry and tone
	Motion	Forehead: none
		Eye: incomplete closure
		Mouth: asymmetry with maximum effort
V		
	Gross	Barely perceptible or no motion
	At rest	Asymmetry
	Motion	Forehead: none

TABLE 1. *Continued*

Grade	Description	
	Eye:	none or incomplete closure
	Mouth:	slight or no movement
VI	No movement. No tone.	

Nervus intermedius function is classified with these suffixes: Crocodile tears, C; C0, no crocodile tears; C1, crocodile tears present. Metallic or aberrant taste, T; T0, no aberrant taste; T1, metallic or aberrant taste present. Dry eye, E; E0, no dry eye; E1, dry eye present
[a] Synkinesis can be assessed by observing the degree of eye closure when the mouth moves or by forcible protrusion of the lips. Synkinesis may include contracture and/or hemifacial spasm

series quote House Grades I–III as satisfactory and House IV–VI as unsatisfactory. Many patients with this grade of facial nerve function are, however, incapacitated with a dry eye or exposure keratitis, and many require a lateral or medial tarsorrhaphy or a gold weight in the upper eyelid. The House-Brackmann grading system also does not take into account nervus intermedius function.

The participants in the consensus meeting discussed the various facial nerve grading systems already in existence and the modification of the House-Brackmann classification proposed by Moffat. In this classification Grade III is subdivided into Grade IIIA and Grade IIIB to take into account the deficiencies in the House-Brackmann system. Grade IIIA is competent eye closure, with the eye comfortable and in good condition with or without lubricants. Grade IIIB is competent eye closure but a dry eye which is uncomfortable, with evidence of exposure keratitis requiring lubricants and possibly tarsorrhaphy.

The degree of synkinesis seen in each of the grades is defined as well as a description of how to elicit it in the test situation. Hemifacial spasm and contracture in relation to synkinesis is also described.

The new classification allows a record of nervus intermedius function with regard to crocodile tears (C), metallic or aberrant taste (T), and dry eye (E). This was finally accepted after alteration, clarification, and the addition of the assessment and degree of synkinesis. Consensus was finally reached on the following classification as described in Table 1.

Session III: Grading Systems for Preoperative and Postoperative Hearing

Mario Sanna[1], Toshimitsu Kobayashi[2], and Jin Kanzaki[3]

Key words. Vestibular schwannoma, Hearing preservation, Preoperative hearing, Postoperative hearing, Hearing classification

Treatment of vestibular schwannoma during the last decade underwent significant advances. The use of sophisticated diagnostic methods such as magnetic resonance imaging (MRI) and auditory bain stun response (ABR) has considerably increased the number of patients diagnosed with small tumors and has restored good (social) hearing. Mortality associated with surgery has become minimal in established centers, and total tumor removal is a rule in most cases. The development of intraoperative monitoring techniques to determine cranial nerve function has considerably decreased the risk of neurological deficit, especially of the facial nerve, in patients with small tumors. Such situations have brought us to the point where the attention of both patients and surgeons can be focused on the issue of hearing preservation.

Various attempts to control vestibular schwannomas, with hearing preservation, are employed; and many articles have been appeared concerning this issue. Preservation of hearing depends highly on the criteria for preserved hearing; and many of the articles concerned with hearing preservation seem to describe hearing that really is not preserved as "preserved." Vestibular schwannoma is a disease, so we believe we must share our experience to advance the cause of learning preservation. We must find the same language in which to dictate, evaluate, and compare our hearing results without misleading others.

[1] Gruppo Otologico, Piacenza, Italy
[2] Department of Otoloryngology, Tohoku University School of Medicine, Sendai, Japan
[3] Department of Otolaryngology, Keio University School of Medicine, Tokyo, Japan

At present, various classification systems are used. The most prevalent currently used classification system includes guidelines for evaluating hearing preservation in patients with acoustic neuroma offered by the American Academy of Otolaryngology–Head and Neck Surgery (AAO) in 1995. However, crucial criticisms of the AAO classification should be raised. First, instead of the commonly used 4000 Hz, it requires measurement of 3000 Hz, which is rarely used in other countries. Second, the classification is too rough, classifying the hearing in only four categories. It classifies 30 dB pure tone average (PTA)/70% speech discrimination score (SDS) as good hearing (class A), and 50 dB PTA/50% SDS as the second best hearing (class B). Because hearing is often impaired after any kind of therapy, such a rough classification increases the chance of reporting significant hearing deterioration as "not changed" or "preserved." This makes the results of hearing preservation therapy look better than it actually is. Third, the classification does not consider normal hearing and really useful hearing when contralateral hearing is normal, which is often the case with a vestibular schwannoma. Here, we must remember that the SDS value is obtained under artificial stimulation. For its measurement, we present a sound markedly above the PTA (e.g., 85 dB), although a 50 dB hearing threshold with 50% SDS in 85 dB (class B in the AAO system) has limited meaning without a hearing aid and very little meaning if the contralateral hearing is normal. Of course, neurofibromatosis type II is not the case. Taking such insufficiencies into consideration, we must find a more detailed classification that agrees with the audiology results and shows the results as they truly are.

We offer some solutions. First, we adopted, on average, 500, 1000, 2000, and 4000 Hz for calculating the PTA. Second, we created a category of "normal" hearing not only for the vestibular schwannoma world but for the real, universal world (i.e., 20 dB PTA and 80% SDS). Third, social hearing should be hearing that can be used even when the contralateral hearing is normal. The limit is 30 dB PTA and 70% SDS. After these two classes, the classification should be as simple and linear as possible, as with Sanna's classification in which PTA and SDS are classified by 20 dB and 20% steps, respectively.

For word recognition, we give more weight to SDS than to PTA. Two measures are thus introduced: (1) Hearing is classified by 10% steps for SDS and by 20 dB steps for PTA. (2) A better SDS class than PTA class makes the category of the patient one class better. The classification is summarized in Table 1, and a nomogram is shown in Fig. 1.

We have reached a consensus that two classes, reflecting normal and social hearing, are needed. However, there has been much discussion about categorizing the hearing after these two classes. Such discussion includes more detailed classification by 10 dB PTA and 10% SDS or by 20 dB and 20% SDS.

TABLE 1. Hearing classification scheme

Class	PTA (dB)	SDS (%)
A	0–20	100–80
B	21–30	79–70
C	31–40	69–60
D	41–60	59–50
E	61–80	49–40
F	81–	39–0

PTA is obtained by averaging four frequencies: 0.5, 1.0, 2.0, and 4.0 kHz. Hearing is classified based on either the PTA or the SDS, whichever is worse. A better SDS class than PTA class causes the category to be one class higher. For example, a patient with 60 dB PTA and 75% SDS is classified as class C

PTA, pure tone average; SDS, speech discrimination score

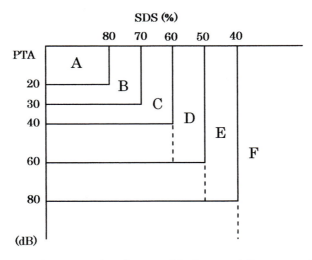

FIG. 1. Nomogram for hearing classification. If the hearing ability crosses the dotted lines, it is designated as being one class higher

The range of 40 dB PTA in class C may be too large, and the dotted line in Fig. 1 might not be necessary. We understand that the classification we present here is not satisfactory, but we believe it is a step toward presenting some solution to an important issue that currently seems to be ignored.

Session IV: Evaluation of Preoperative Symptoms and Postoperative Complications

Takanori Fukushima[1] and Tomio Sasaki[2]

Key words. Acoustic neuroma, Dizziness, Vertigo, Tinnitus, Dysequilibrium

Introduction

Advances in diagnostic neuroimaging and microsurgical technical skills have facilitated accurate and safe operative management of acoustic neuromas. Currently, total tumor removal can be achieved in most cases, with negligible mortality and morbidity. However, some of the general surgical complications, such as wound infection, cerebiospinal fluid (CSF) leak, or meningitis, may occur, as may worsening of preoperative symptoms. There was singificant discussion at the international consensus meeting about evaluating and assessing the degree of preoperative symptoms and postoperative complications. A method to evaluate preoperative symptoms and postoperative sequelae other than hearing deficits and facial nerve weakness is presented in this chapter.

Preoperative Symptoms

Dizziness and tinnitus are the most common preoperative symptoms in patients with an acoustic neuroma. There have been a number of clinical papers regarding the assessment of pre- and postoperative tinnitus. Considering the fact that dizziness and tinnitus are subjective symptoms, such symptoms should be graded by a simple classification system that includes precise

[1] Carolina Neuroscience Institute, 4030 Wake Forest Road, Suite 115, Raleigh, NC 27529, USA
[2] Department of Neurosurgery, Gumma University Medical School, Gumma, Japan

history taking. After a full range of discussion among specialists, the following simple grading system has been adopted for the evaluation of tinnitus.

Grade I: no tinnitus
Grade II: occasional or slight tinnitus
Grade III: moderate, constant tinnitus that is annoying but tolerable
Grade IV: constant, severe tinnitus that bothers the patient and disturbs work or sleep

Similarly, dizziness, vertigo, or dysequilibrium should be classified using the following simple grading system.

Grade I: normal, no dizziness
Grade II: occasional or slight dizziness
Grade III: moderate and frequent dizziness or vertigo
Grade IV: frequent or constant severe dizziness and vertigo, incapacitating the patients in terms of daily life activities

Postoperative Complications

Postoperative symptoms and complications are classified into three categories: temporary complications, permanent symptoms, and permanent objective deficits.

Temporary complications
    Cranial nerve deficit (III–X)
    Dysequilibrium or ataxia
    Hemiparesis
    Hemorrhage
    Hematomas
    Stroke
    Infarction
    CSF leak
    Meningitis
    Wound infection
    Hydrocephalus
Permanent subjective symptoms
    Dizziness, vertigo, and dysequilibrium
    Tinnitus
    Chronic headache
Permanent objective deficits
    Ataxia
    Fine movement disorders (dysdiadochokinesis)

Hemiparesis
Trigeminal facial hypesthesia
Diplopia
Dysphagia, hoarseness
Speech disturbance
Mental disturbance
Seizure disorder

Each postoperative symptom and deficit listed above can be evaluated uniformly using the following grading system.

Grade I: no symptoms or deficits
Grade II: slight symptoms or slight deficit
Grade III: moderate problems or moderate deficit
Grade IV: severe problems and major deficit

There were a number of discussions and controversies among specialists while simplifying and standardizing the evaluation of the postoperative problems. The simple and easily understandable grading systems noted here have been approved and are easily applicable for both neurosurgeons and neurootologists.

Session V: Evaluation of the Effect of Radiotherapy

Jacques P.Y. Magnan[1] and Yuichi Inoue[2]

When faced with a patient with an acoustic neuroma we have three options [1]: wait and scan, radiotherapy, surgery. All of these options require a clear assessment with the same accuracy and the same criteria.

Marseille, the second largest city in France (after Paris), is the only center to have used gamma knife surgery for the past 10 years. Even with this record, however, it is difficult to obtain accurate information on the follow-up of these patients. The presentations are always a mixture of clinical reports and advertising, with modifications of the doses and the follow-up periods. When the gamma knife was first used in Marseille [2], the indication was the presence of a small or medium-sized tumor (1–2 cm) in the cerebillopontine angle (CPA). Such tumors were treated with 18–20 Gy marginal doses.

Nowadays [3,4] there is a trend to extend the indications to intracanalicular tumors and to tumors larger than 30 mm but to apply lower doses (11–14 Gy) to minimize the side effects.

The literature reflects this change, with each proponent promoting his or her own attitude, claiming [5,6] a high percentage of good results and a low incidence of side effects, only to be challenged by the competitors [7–10].

In 2001 Kaylie et al. [11] said: "Surgery remains the treatment of choice for most tumors until alternative therapies, such as gamma knife, use uniform grading scales and show long term facial and hearing results." At the same time Andrews et al. [12] concluded that: "at 1-year follow-up, a significantly higher rate of serviceable hearing preservation was achieved in fractionated SRT (fractionated stereotactic radiotherapy) sporadic tumor patients,

[1] Professor of Aix-Marseille II University, ORL-Hospital Nord, 13915 Marseille, Credex 20, France
[2] Department of Radiology, School of Medicine, Osaka City University, Osaka, Japan

and may therefore be preferable to alternatives including surgery, SRS (sterotactic radiosurgery) or possibly observation in patients with serviceable hearing." This assertion was condemned in advance by Linskey [13] in 2000: "a disturbing trend is developing in which institutions without non-gamma-knife radiosurgery (GKS) centers are championing and/or shifting to hypofractionated sterotactic radiotherapy for vestibular schwannomas. Aggressive advertising and marketing from some of these centers even paradoxically suggests biological superiority of hypofractionation approaches over single-dose radiosurgery for vestibular schwannomas."

At present, we accept Kaylie et al.'s conclusion [14] as our own: "Surgery on all sized tumors has a significantly lower complication rate than radiosurgery peformed on tumors smaller than 4 cm ($P = 3.2 \times 10$)" [14]. Surgery has a lower major morbidity rate than gamma knife radiosurgery ($P = 2.4 \times 10$) [14]. Tumor control is defined as no tumor recurrence or regrowth. Surgery offers superior tumor control when tumors are totally resected ($P = 9.02 \times 10$) [11]. Assuming that all partially resected tumors recur, surgery retains a significant advantage over radiosurgery for tumor control ($P = 0.028$).

Data from these studies date back to the late 1960s and do not completely reflect outcomes using current imaging and procedures. A major difficulty encountered is the inconsistent data reporting. Future surgical and irradiation reports should use standardized outcome scales to allow valid statistical comparisons. In addition, there have been no reported long-term results from gamma knife radiosurgery using lower dosimetry. Surgery should remain the therapy of choice for acoustic neuromas until tumor control rates can be established."

It is at this point we now find ourselves. During this session it was outside our field of endeavor to discuss the advantages or disadvantages of radiotherapy for acoustic neuromas. Our goal was only to find a better way to evaluate the effect of radiotherapy and consequently to be able to compare the results between surgery and radiotherapy.

It is relevant to start with definitions so we speak the same language. Then we can discuss and present our conclusions on the following three questions.

1. *How do we evaluate the effect of radiotherapy using tumor size follow-up grading?* The proposed classification consists of three groups.

Grade 1: Tumor is controlled, that is, the tumor shrinks >2 mm (tumor size should be evaluated using the largest dimension of the CPA) or the volume is decreased by 10%, calculated by computer mapping.

Grade 2: Tumor is stabilized, that is, there is no change in tumor size (< to 2 mm>) or volume (< to 10% >). The designation "tumor control" cannot be used for grade 2 lesions owing to the natural course of the disease.

Grade 3: Tumor is progressing, that is, the tumor is now > 2 mm in largest dimension or its volume is increasing.

Imaging must be performed each year.

2. *How do we describe the various kinds of radiosurgery?* Radiosurgery consists of the delivery of a single fraction in a small volume but a high dose of radiation to the brain such as by gamma knife or Xknife. Stereotactic radiotherapy delivers a multiple-fraction, hyperdose of therapeutic radiation, such as by the fractionated linear accelerator technique (LINAC).

3. *How do we evaluate the sequelae of radiotherapy?* The sequelae of radiotherapy must be evaluated in the same way, with the same grading system regarding pre- and postoperative symptoms. The items to be evaluated are: facial nerve function, hearing preservation, tinnitus, unsteadinness, and neuropathological problems.

References

1. Moller P, Myreseth E, Pedersen PH, Larsen JL, Krakenes J, Moen G (2000) Acoustic neuroma—treatment modalities: surgery, gamma knife or observation? Acta Otolaryngol 543(suppl):34–37
2. Regis J, Pellet W (1998) Radiosurgery or microsurgery of vestibular schwannomas. Cancer Radiother 2:191–201
3. Flickinger JC, Kondziolka D, Pollock BE, Lunsford LD (1996) Evolution in technique for vestibular schwannoma radiosurgery and effect on outcome. Int J Radiat Oncol Biol Phys 36:275–288
4. Niranjan A, Lunsford LD, Flickinger JC, Maitz A, Kondziolka D (1999) Dose reduction improves hearing preservation rates after intracanalicular acoustic tumor radiosurgery. Neurosurgery 45:753–762
5. Pollock BE, Lunsford LD, Noren G (1998) Vestibular schwannoma management in the next century: a radiosurgical perspective. Neurosurgery 43:475–481
6. Sims E, Doughty D, Macaulay E, Royle N, Wraith C, Darlinson R, Plowman PN (1999) Stereotactically delivered cranial radiation therapy: a ten-year experience of linac-based radiosurgery in the UK. Clin Oncol 11:303–320
7. Yamamoto M, Ide M, Umebara S, Jimbo M, Takakura K (1996) Gamma knife radiosurgery for brain tumors: post irradiation volume changes compared with preradiosurgical growth fractions. Neurol Med Chir (Tokyo) 36:358–363
8. Hanabus K, Morikawa A, Murata T, Taki W (2001) Acoustic neuroma with malignant transformation case report. J Neurosurg 95:518–521
9. Thomsen J, Mirz F, Wetke R, Astrup J, Bojsen-Moller M, Nielsen E (2000) Intracranial sarcoma in a patient with neurofibromatosis type 2 treated with gamma knife radiosurgery for vestibular schwannoma. Am J Otol 21:364–370
10. Luetje CM (2000) Spontaneous involution of acoustic tumors. Am J Otol 21:393–398
11. Kaylie DM, Gilbert E, Horgan MA, Delashaw JB, McMenomey SO (2001) Acoustic neuroma surgery outcomes. Otol Neurootol 22:686–689
12. Andrews DW, Suarez O, Goldman HW, et al (2001) Stereotactic radiosurgery and fractionated stereotatic radiotherapy for the treatment of acoustic schwannomas: comparatives observations of 125 patients treated at one institution. Int J Radiat Oncol Biol Phys 50:1265–1278

13. Linskey ME (2000) Stereotactic radiosurgery versus stereotactic radiotherapy for patients with vestibular schwannoma: a Leksell Gamma Knife Society 2000 debate. J Neurosurg 93(suppl 3):90–95
14. Kaylie DM, Horgan MJ, Delashaw JB, McMenomey SO (2000) A meta-analysis comparing outcomes of microsurgery and gamma knife radiosurgery. Laryngoscope 110: 1850–1856

Session VI: Other Issues

Bruce J. Gantz[1] and Masaru Aoyagi[2]

1. Repaired facial nerve recovery grading system
    a. Recognize it is difficult to use the House-Brackmann classification to report functional results when a facial nerve has undergone repair
    b. Iowa Repaired Facial Nerve Recovery Scale [1]
2. Objective facial nerve grading systems
    a. Promising for the future
    b. Continue to study
3. Cystic nature of tumors
    a. Identify as separate group
    b. Consider cystic if there are cysts or multiple cysts on the surface of the tumor
4. Adhesion of tumor
    a. Unable to measure; highly subjective
5. Vascularity of tumor
    a. Unable to measure; highly subjective

Repair of the facial nerve is not a common procedure performed in the present era of microsurgery for acoustic neuroma. When the facial nerve has been disrupted, repair can be performed using primary anastomosis of the nerve or an interposition nerve graft. Both strategies reestablish the integrity of the facial nerve and can provide strong closure of the eye and mouth, as well as some mimetic function. Generally, mass motion is apparent, and movement of the temporal branch of the nerve is rare. For this reason, functional recovery graded by facial motion is difficult using the House-

[1] Professor and Head Brian F. McCabe Distinguished Chair in Otolaryngology-Head and Neck Surgery The University of Iowa Hospitals and Clinics 200 Hawkins Drive, Iowa City IA 52242-1078, USA
[2] Professor, Department of Otolaryngology, School of Medicine, Yamagata University, Yamagata, Japan

Brackmann (H-B) facial nerve grading system. According to the H-B criteria, the best score for a repaired nerve would be grade IV/VI because of the mass motion, synkinesis, and lack of forehead movement. In reality, repairs result in strong eye closure, wheseas H-B IV recovery indicates incomplete eye closure. For these reasons a separate grading system for repaired facial nerves is required. It is the consensus of the group that the Iowa Repaired Facial Nerve Recovery Scale [1] should be used to grade facial function following repair of the facial nerve.

It is the impression of the consensus group that multicystic tumors present challenging surgical problems and are generally difficult to remove. To study this phenomenon it is recommended that multicystic tumors be identified as a separate entity when reporting results. Tumors to be included in this group are those in which the cystic components are on the surface of the tumor. Central cystic components of solid tumors should not be included in this grouping.

Other aspects of the tumor, including firmness, vascularity, and the "stickiness" or adhesive nature of the tumor, cannot be measured. Hence they should not be included in the description of results.

Finally, objective grading systems for postoperative facial motor function are in development. Several systems were demonstrated, and continued development of these systems is encouraged. There is insufficient experience with any system to recommend a specific protocol at this time.

Reference

1. Gidley PW, Gantz BJ, Rubinstein JT (1999) Facial nerve grafts: from cerebello-pontine angle and beyond. Am J Otol 20:781–788

Appendix: Results of Questionnaires of Reporting System

JIN KANZAKI

Questionnaire Respondents

Altogether, 10 European, 10 U.S., and 6 Asian surgeons responded to the questionnaires (before consensus meeting).

The surgeons who responded were J. Magnan (France), M. Wigand (Germany), J. Helms (Germany), O. Sterkers (France), M. Tos (Denmark), J. Thomsen (Denmark), U. Fisch (Switzerland), B. Gantz (USA), T. Fukushima (USA), M. Aristegui (Spain), R. Charachon (France), L. Shekar (USA), A. Mazzoni (Italy), C. Kim (Korea), A. Hakuba (Japan), S. Hashimoto (Japan), S. Kobayashi (Japan), S. Murakami (Japan), and K. Ishikawa (Japan).

The institutions that responded were the House Institute (seven surgeons) and the Japan Society of Acoustic Neuroma.

Tumor Size

In Europe the diameter of a tumor in the cerebellopontine angle (CPA) in the direction parallel to the internal auditory canal (IAC) (a) and $a \times b$ (diameter perpendicular to the IAC) has been used primarily, whereas those in the United States have mostly adopted use of the diameter of the IAC + CPA (a) and $(a + c) \times b$. In Asia, $a \times b$ and root $a \times b$ are mainly used. (The Japan Society of Acoustic Neuroma has adopted $a \times b$.)

For intracanalicular lesions, tumor size is expressed by its diameter in the direction of the IAC; if there is space in the fundus lateral to a tumor, the space is measured and is shown as "d mm from the fundus" or "d mm + fundus space (mm)."

Department of Otolaryngology, School of Medicine, Keio University, Tokyo, Japan

For tumors extending to the CPA the size of a lesion is shown as its largest extracanalicular dimension (or its situation is described) or as the CPA diameter + intracanicular distance (from the fundus). The term "medial tumor" is used by some for a tumor that is not in the IAC.

Classification

There are various classifications of the tumors (e.g., small, medium, large, giant). In fact, there are 12 classifications offered by 11 surgeons.

Preoperative and Postoperative Hearing

The results of preoperative and postoperative hearing are mainly reported according to the AAO-HNS classification. There are, however, other systems, such as those of Shelton, Gardner, and Sanna, that are used in both Europe and the United States. Postoperative evaluation is done at various intervals, but it is mainly at 6 months postoperatively in the United States and at 12 months in Europe.

Facial Nerve Function

Facial nerve function is evaluated mostly by the House-Brackmann method, although a grading system developed in their own country seems to be used there. Postoperative evaluation is usually done 12 months after surgery but occasionally at 3 or 6 months.

【 Results of Questionnaires / Session I 】

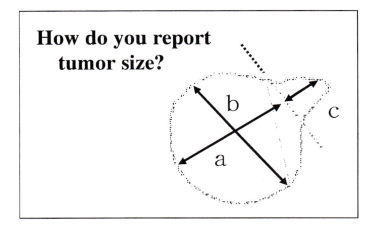

Table 1.

Answer	Europe (n=10)	USA (n=10)	Asia (n=6)
a	3		
a+c	1	4	
a×b	2		3
(a+c)×b	1	4	
√ab		1	3
a or b	2		
√d(a+c)b d.vertical diameter		1	
Largest diameter	1	1※	

※Multiple answers

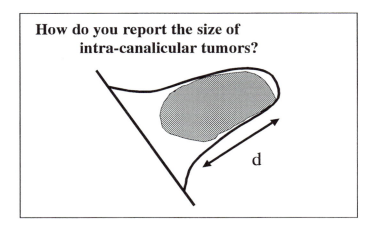

Table 2.

Answer	Europe (n=10)	USA (n=10)	Asia (n=6)
d mm	6	10	6
descriptive	2		
d + fundus space	1		
d mm from fundus	1		

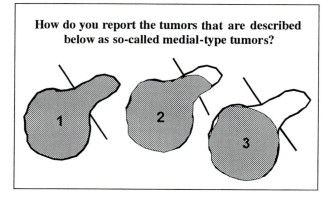

How do you report the tumors that are described below as so-called medial-type tumors?

Table 3.

Answer	Europe (n=10)	USA (n=9)	Asia (n=6)
1+2+3			
1) IAC+CPA staging	1		
2) largest extra-canalicular diameter	1		
3) descriptive	2	5	1
4) CPA diameter + IC diameter from fundus	1	3	
Only 3	4	1	5
Does not exist	1		

If you report tumor size as small, medium, large, or giant, how do you define each size?

Table 4-a.

Europe

	Classification 1	Classification 2	Classification 3
Small	0−15	0−10	1−10
Medium	16−25	10−25	11−20
Large	26−40	25−40	21−30
Giant	41<	40<	31<

(mm)

Table 4-b.

Europe

	Classification 4	Classification 5	Classification 6
Small	0−20	0−19	10−12
Medium	20−40	20−29	13−25
Large	40<	30−39	25−35
Giant		40<	35<

(mm)

Table 4 - c.

USA

	Classification 1	Classification 2	Classification 3
Small	0−15	0−10	5−15
Medium	15−25	10−25	15−29
Large	25−40	25−35	30−40
Giant	40<	35<	41−60

(mm)

Table 4-d.

USA

	Classification 4	Classification 5	Classification 6
Small	0−20	1−9	3−14
Medium	21−40	10−24	15−24
Large	40<	25−39	25−34
Giant		40<	35−70

(mm)

Table 4-e.

Asia

	Classification 1	Classification 2	Classification 3
Small	5−15	1−15	0−10
Medium	15−25	16−30	11−30
Large	25−50	31−40	31−40
Giant	50<	41<	41<

(mm)

Asia

Table 4-f.

	Classification 4	Classification 5	Classification 6
Small	0–10	0–10	0–10
Medium	11–30	10–20	11–25
Large	31–50	20–30	25–40
Giant	51<	30<	41<

(mm)

How do you define total removal, subtotal removal, and partial removal of a tumor ?

[Total removal]

Table 5-a.

	Europe (n=9)	USA (n=10)	Asia (n=6)
100% +complete removal	8	9	4
Post-op MRI		1	
No tumor at the end of surgery and at 3 years post-op	1		
Other description			2

[Near-total removal]

Table 5-b.

	Europe (n=8)	USA (n=10)	Asia (n=6)
90% <		3	2
98% <		2	
99% <	2		2
Very small pieces	4	3	2
Sheet of arachnoid on facial nerve	1		
Tumor matrix	1		
Do not use		2	

[Subtotal removal]

Table 5-c.

	Europe (n=9)	USA (n=8)	Asia (n=6)
Descriptive + MRI	2	2	
< 99%, > 90%	3	3	3
< 90%, > 50%		1	1
Others	4	2	2

[Partial removal]

Table 5-d.

	Europe (n=6)	USA (n=5)	Asia (n=6)
100−50%	2		
< 90%	1	1	2
< 75%	2	1	
< 50%		1	1
Others	1	2	3

【 Results of Questionnaires / Session II 】

How do you report pre- and post-operative facial nerve function?

Table 1.

Grading system	Europe (n=9)	USA (n=10)	Asia (n=6)
House-Brackmann	8	10	5※
Yanagihara			2※
Stennert	2 ※		
Fisch	1		1
Objective	1 ※		

(※ Overlapping)

When should post-operative facial nerve function be evaluated?

Table 2.

Post-op evaluation	Europe (n=9)	USA (n=10)	Asia (n=6)
6, 12 months		3	1
12 months	7	4	3
3, 12 months		1	1
Immediate—at discharge 12 months		1	
Immediate		1	
18 months	1		
12 months + 24 months	1		
Depends on tumor size			1

【 Results of Questionnaires / Session Ⅲ 】

How do you report
pre- and post-operative hearing?

According to:

Table 1.

Classification	Europe (n=11)	USA (n=9)	Asia (n=6)
AAO-HNS	5	6	4
Shelton	2	1	2
Gardner	2	1	
Sanna	2		
(not specified)		1	

When should post-operative hearing be evaluated?

Table 2.

Post-op evaluation	Europe (n=9)	USA (n=9)	Asia (n=6)
6 months		4	4
1, 6, and 12 months	1		
6, 12 months		1	1
1, 6 months		1	
3 months, 1 year and 2 years		1	
Immediate, 1, 3 months and 1 year		1	
12 months	6	1	1
1 week , 6-12 weeks and 1 year	1		
1 , 3 , 12 and 36 months	1		

Key Word Index